H

Herb

Healing with Herbs and Rituals

A MEXICAN TRADITION

Eliseo "Cheo" Torres
Edited by Timothy L. Sawyer, Jr.

UNIVERSITY OF NEW MEXICO PRESS | ALBUQUERQUE

©2006 by the University of New Mexico Press
All rights reserved. Published 2006
Printed in the United States of America

12   11   10   09   08   07   06   1   2   3   4   5   6   7

LIBRARY OF CONGRESS CATALOGING-IN-PUBLICATION DATA

Torres, Eliseo.
  Healing with herbs and rituals : a Mexican tradition / Eliseo "Cheo" Torres ;
edited by Timothy L. Sawyer, Jr.
    p. cm.
  This volume is a combination with revisions of two of the author's earlier
works entitled Folk healer and Green medicine.
  Includes index.
  ISBN-13: 978-0-8263-3961-4 (pbk. : alk. paper)
  ISBN-10: 0-8263-3961-1 (pbk. : alk. paper)
  1. Herbs—Therapeutic use—Mexico. 2. Traditional medicine—Mexico.
3. Mexican Americans—Medicine. 4. Healers—Mexico. 5. Healing—Mexico.
I. Torres, Eliseo. Folk healer. II. Torres, Eliseo. Green medicine.
III. Sawyer, Timothy L. (Timothy Leighton), 1961– IV. Title.
  RM666.H33.T672 2006
  615'.321—dc22

                              2005025893

DESIGN AND COMPOSITION: MELISSA TANDYSH

About the cover: The photos (*from top to bottom*) are of Don Pedrito Jaramillo,
Nino Fidencio, and Teresita, three great curanderos of Mexico and the
Southwest.

Contents

Preface to Current Edition

The current volume is a combination of the two earlier books into a single work. Rather than continue to self-publish, I have decided to bring my research and experiences to a wider audience by publishing with an established and respected academic publisher, the University of New Mexico Press. The division of the current volume into two separate sections reflects the old division of separate works that preceded this one, i.e. Part One is *Folk Healer* (renamed here "Folk Healers and Folk Healing") and Part Two is *Green Medicine* (titled here "Green Medicine: Traditional Mexican-American Herbs and Remedies").

I have also added new herbs to Part Two of the book and have listed botanical names wherever possible. Please be aware that some of the herbs listed are inexactly identified in the literature and tradition, and that sometimes a broad term, like "pine," is difficult to pinpoint as to the exact species used for a particular remedy. The botanical names will sometimes reflect this imprecision.

Part One

*Folk Healers
and Folk Healing*

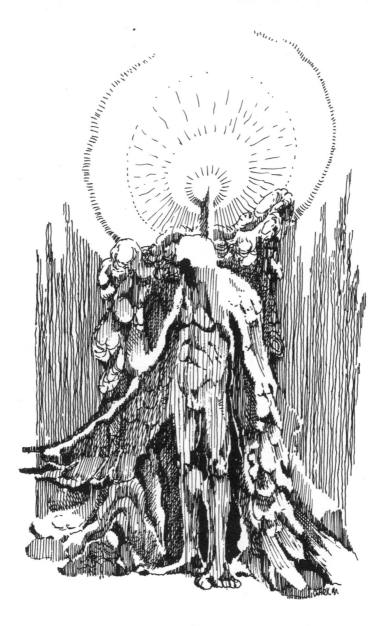

Figure 1: Candles are used in rituals and the flame, color, and shape of each is significant in healing or in attracting certain powers.

Introduction

Even as a child growing up in a small community, I was fascinated by the practice of *curanderismo,* or folk healing. I vividly remember the ritual to cure *mal de ojo*—the evil eye—with its prayers and the use of the egg. There were days that I would have a mild *cólico* (stomachache) and would get the treatment for that. Also, there were many times that I would experience a bad fright and suffer from *susto* and have to be spiritually cleansed with a broom, that is, swept with branches of rue, or *ruda.* Still, though I grew up with it, it is difficult to explain, not so much the rituals of curanderismo, but the love and the faith associated with it.

Nonetheless, I wanted to try. I felt it was very important to keep curanderismo alive, and also to acquaint the general public with its importance in the Mexican and Mexican-American culture. I began to do this while I was still a doctoral student.

At first I concentrated on the herbs. It was natural to begin here, remembering as I did that for every illness and with every ritual there would always be a freshly brewed cup of tea: perhaps chamomile (*manzanilla*), mint (*yerba buena*), or aniseed (*anís*). During visits to relatives or friends, cuttings of different varieties of plants that were used to make the teas were always given to my mother, who quickly got them into the earth once we got home!

With this in mind, I developed a teaching unit on Folk Medicine and Medicinal Herbs of the Southwest and Northern Mexico. I interviewed several *curanderos*—folk healers—and *yerberos*—herbalists—in Mexican towns and in towns in the Rio Grande Valley and along the border in the United States. After that, I gave many lectures, in person and on television, about the subject.

It became clear that interest in curanderismo was high, and yet available works on the subject—particularly works aimed at the average person rather than the sociologist or scholar—were few and far between. I felt I had to expand my lecture notes into something more substantial to fill this need.

So that is how my first book, *Green Medicine: Traditional Mexican-American Herbal Remedies*, came into being. From there, it seemed only natural to go on to describe the practices surrounding the use of those herbs—the same rituals that I recall from my childhood. Thus I was led to prepare a companion volume, *Folk Healer: The Mexican-American Tradition of Curanderismo*. These two books are now updated and combined into this publication.

Chapter One

A Brief History of Curanderismo

The term curanderismo may be translated "folk healing." A *curandero* or *curandera*, then, is a healer, with the letter at the end of the word signifying whether male or female. All three words derive from the Spanish verb *curar*, which means to heal.

The roots of curanderismo are many. The Moors, for instance, brought in Arabic elements, which came to the New World via Spain. The theory of "the humors," with its emphasis on balance between light and darkness, heat and cold, was introduced this way. Some beliefs associated with curanderismo, particularly the insistence that all power to heal comes from God, are Biblical and therefore Judeo-Christian in origin. And, of course, there are powerful Indian—particularly Aztec—influences, too, most often in the herbal remedies that are used.

Curanderismo has always embraced three levels, though certain curanderos may choose to emphasize one above—or even to the exclusion of—the others. These are the material (the most common, with emphasis on objects such as candles, oils, herbs), the spiritual (here the curandero is often a medium), and the mental (psychic healers, for example). Rituals—formulaic or patterned ways of treating the various illnesses of those who come to see the curandero—are performed on all three levels.

One needn't be familiar with curanderismo nor believe in it in order for it to work. Evelyne Winter, in *Mexico's Ancient and Native Remedies*, collected this story from a woman named Muriel Balfour. Mrs. Balfour's husband had obviously been treated by a curandero, but—just as obvious—the Balfours had no idea that this was so, nor that the treatment given was pretty much "standard operating procedure" in curanderismo. The point is, though the Balfour's were not predisposed to believe, the cure worked! Here is Mrs. Balfour's account:

> My late husband one time had a very bad eye and headache. A man came to see him to cure him. This "doctor" asked me for a raw egg which I gave him. While the egg was still in its shell he passed it many times over my husband's head and face. Then he asked me for a dish and he opened the egg which had become hard boiled. We asked if it had cured him and he said not entirely. The "doctor" came the next day and went through the same procedure with a fresh egg but after the treatment the egg was not hard boiled, only coddled. The "doctor" was not satisfied that the cure had been completed and came the third day. The egg the third day was unchanged by the treatment and the man pronounced him cured. And my husband *was* cured.

The use of the egg is quite common in curanderismo, perhaps because, as scholars Robert T. Trotter II and Juan Antonio Chavira note in their book, *Curanderismo*, "The material properties of the egg include its ordinary use as food; its mystical properties, however,

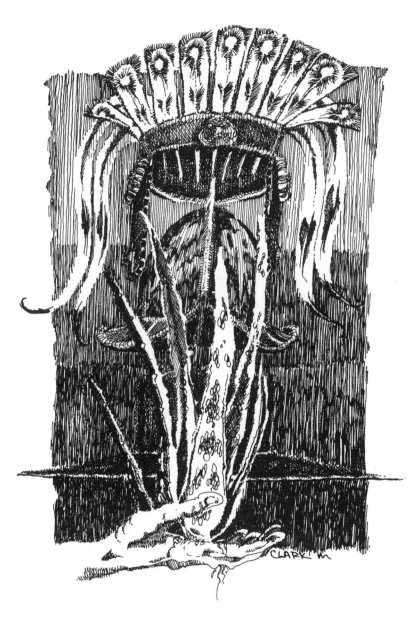

Figure 2: Aloe vera (*zabila*) was introduced by
Spanish missionaries to Native Americans.

include its ability to absorb negative influences (sickness) from a patient." Still another reason is that many rituals demand a sacrificial object, and according to Trotter and Chavira, "the egg qualifies as an animal cell."

In addition to the egg, the lemon figures in the rituals of curanderismo, as does *agua preparada*—specially prepared water. Water, especially water that has been blessed (holy water), is considered a physical link with the spiritual world. In fact, it is not uncommon for a curandero to dip the other objects he is using into holy water to enhance their curative powers.

Fire, too, in the form of candles and incense, plays a part in many of the ceremonies, as do many herbs (see Part Two, Green Medicine) and aromatic oils.

But, as with lemon and the egg, curanderismo also relies on items that are very ordinary indeed. Purple onion, for instance, and garlic are often used. These items are said to protect, while the aforementioned egg and lemon are thought to actually absorb negative forces.

Chapter Two

The Curandero

I t is the state of consciousness that distinguishes the curandero working on the material level: he is awake rather than in a trance and is himself—that is, has not assumed the being of another.

Curanderos also have specialties. A *yerbero* is an herbalist, able to prescribe botanical remedies. A *partera* is a midwife. A *sobador* or *sobadora* is a masseuse or masseur. The three levels of curanderismo touching and crossing each other can easily be seen when we use the *sobador* as an example.

A *sobador* might work only on the material level, using his hands and perhaps an aromatic oil or a poultice or even a tea. But a *sobador* might also heal an illness that exists deep beneath the surface of the skin—indeed, perhaps in the nervous system or in the mind. That *sobador* might be said to operate on the psychic level as well. There are *sobadores*, for instance, who have been said to cure paralysis.

A *señora*, however, because she reads cards in order to foretell the future or reveal the influence of the past, can be said to emphasize the mental or psychic level. An *espiritista* or medium would work entirely on the spiritual level.

While it is true that most curanderos work on the material level, the spiritual mode is growing in popularity. This is particularly due to the *Fidencistas,* followers of Niño Fidencio, a Mexican healer. These followers are said to assume Niño's spirit now that he is dead—that is, *become* him, in order to heal.

Is belief in curanderismo a religious belief, or is it a belief in the supernatural? Well, it is often both. The aforementioned belief that all healing power comes from God makes it religious, as does the very prevalent idea that a curandero can only bring about God's will. The belief that certain rituals or practices can effect a certain outcome is, however, a belief in the supernatural—that is, a belief that outside forces can be changed, controlled. In this way, curanderismo partakes of both the religious and the supernatural. In fact, a curandero can be a *brujo*—a witch—capable of casting evil spells! Curanderismo, therefore, is careful to distinguish between white magic and black magic, with most curanderos espousing the former.

How does one become a curandero? Often—as you will see when you read the stories of the most famous healers—it is a matter of recognizing that one has the God-given gift—the *don*, as it is called. Sometimes, too, it is the result of a long apprenticeship. Many curanderos renounce steady jobs in order to work as healers.

In defining who is and who isn't a curandero, the amount of time one spends healing is usually considered. While most cities and barrios within cities have someone whom they call upon to prescribe teas and other herbal remedies for minor ills, the curandero handles more serious cases. The curandero does not have another job; healing is the basis of the curandero's livelihood.

In the past, another consideration when measuring the authenticity of a given person's claim to being a curandero was whether or not that person charged for his services. The true curandero was said to take what had been offered, and there are many recorded instances, too, of curanderos refusing to accept even small payments when these were offered by the very poor.

Now that is not always the case. When KPRC-TV in Houston did a mini-documentary on two modern curanderos, for instance,

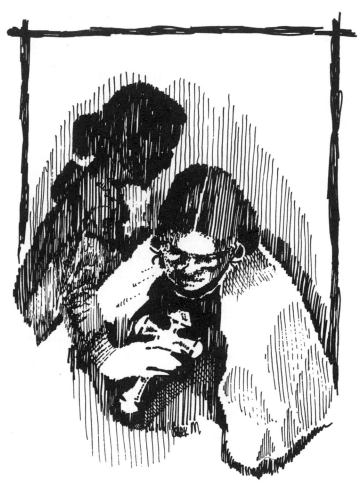

Figure 3: A curandero uses a holistic approach to religion and incorporates religion as well as supernatural beliefs.

they found that the youngest, a woman named María, not only charged for her services, but had an hourly rate. "I charge ten dollars for one hour," María boasted. "What I really should be charging is a hundred and fifty dollars an hour . . . 'cause I'm damn good!"

In many cases, the fact that money is not needed is one reason curanderismo still thrives in Mexican and Mexican-American neighborhoods. Other reasons are that there is no language barrier, no need for an appointment, and, frequently, no necessity to travel great distances. Also, a curandero does not require that his patients have medical insurance or that they fill out complicated forms.

Equally important is the fact that the curandero treats many ailments not even recognized by the formal medical establishment. In many cases, these ailments reflect the patient's psychological state. As Ari Kiev, an author and psychiatrist, has pointed out, curanderismo is a system of medicine that recognizes the profound effect that the emotions can have on health. It takes into account the physical manifestations of such feelings as anger, sorrow, shame, rejection, fear, desire, and disillusionment. When one considers that the holistic movement is the one arm of formal medicine that has finally begun to recognize this, the centuries-old practice of curanderismo seems advanced indeed.

What is formal medicine's attitude toward curanderismo? Well, as you might guess, curanderismo was long regarded as superstition or medicine that, at best, treated only imagined ills. Now, however, the medical establishment has become more tolerant. Again, the holistic movement has done much to promote (for the most part, inadvertently) acceptance of this ancient system. In any case, a lot of writing about curanderismo is addressed to health care professionals and urges them to think of curanderismo as either an alternative or a supplement to formal medicine.

Chapter Three

Ailments

The most common ailments treated by curanderismo are mal de ojo (evil eye), sometimes referred to as *mal ojo*, or just plain *ojo*; as well as *susto* (magical fright); *caída de mollera* (fallen fontanelle); and *empacho* (stomach blockage).

There are also a number of ailments less frequently encountered, and these would be found in Mexico more often than in the United States. These are *mal aire* (respiratory infection), sometimes just called *aire*; *desasombro* (high level of susto); *espanto* (serious loss of spirit); *bilis* (suppressed anger); *muína* (rage); and *latido* (nervous stomach).

Then, too, there are ills brought about by evil or witchcraft. These are *envidia*, *mal puesto*, *salar*, and *maleficio*.

Definitions of the various ailments and their causes differ, but those that follow are generally accepted.

Mal de ojo
Although this sounds as though it is inflicted through malice, the opposite is the case. Mal de ojo—the evil eye—comes about through

excessive admiration, usually of those too weak to absorb it. Babies are the most frequent victims, but animals can contract ojo, too. Charms are worn by those susceptible to evil eye. The most common is an adorned seed resembling a deer's eye called *ojo de venado*.

Why would admiration cause illness? Some scholars say that it arises from the belief that a person projects something of himself when he admires another. If the person receiving the admiration can't handle it, either because of youth or weakness, illness results.

To counteract the effect of the admiration and guard against mal de ojo, the admirer must touch the person, animal, or object of his admiration.

The symptoms of ojo are similar to those of colic: irritability, drooping eyes, fever, headache, and vomiting.

Susto

Sometimes susto is translated as loss of spirit or even loss of soul. Occasionally, it is translated as shock, though it shouldn't be confused with the life-threatening medical condition known as shock. A common definition is fright, or magical fright.

Receiving bad news can cause susto, as can any bad scare. It is thought that such a scare can temporarily drive the person's spirit or soul from the body. Susto has to be treated immediately or it will lead to the much more serious *susto pasado* or, in Mexico, *susto meco*—an old susto that is much more difficult to treat and can lead to death.

Weakness is a symptom of susto. Or, as Dolores Latorre describes it in *Cooking and Curing With Mexican Herbs*, "the victim suddenly feels wobbly, chilly, shaky, limp, and drowsy, or he may develop a headache accompanied by nausea." On the other hand, when Ari Kiev describes the symptoms in *Curanderismo*, he writes that they are "a mixture of anxiety—dyspnea, indigestion, palpitations, and depression—loss of interest in things, irritability, insomnia, and anorexia." Kiev relates one curandero's belief that a susto untreated can lead to heart attack.

Caída de mollera

This condition—in English known as "fallen fontanelle"—afflicts only babies. The symptoms are irritability, diarrhea, and vomiting. The baby thus becomes dehydrated and exhibits the most prominent symptom, the one that gives the condition its name: a depressed fontanelle (soft spot).

Caída de mollera is thought to be caused by rough handling or from pulling the baby's bottle or the mother's breast from his mouth while he is nursing. It can also, however, be caused by a fall from the bed or crib. Or the baby can cause it himself by sucking too greedily.

Empacho

The main symptom of this ill is diarrhea and a feeling of weight in the pit of one's stomach. Loss of appetite (not surprisingly) follows.

The symptoms of empacho are thought to be produced by something actually stuck in the stomach or blocking the intestines. It can afflict adults, but children are the usual victims.

Empacho is an ailment that reflects the need for balance that is expressed in the theory of the humors—that is, it is thought to be caused by improperly mixing hot with cold foods, or eating such foods in improper sequence. Eating too quickly and thus not chewing food completely is another act thought to cause empacho.

As an interesting side note, Ari Kiev points out that both empacho and caída de mollera "are associated with the proper management of children" and are therefore ailments whose presence arouses feelings of guilt in the parents.

Mal aire

This seems similar to an upper respiratory infection in that it produces earache, stiff neck, chills, dizziness, and headache. Often called "a cold," this ailment can be referred to as aire.

Desasombro

Desasombro is thought to be a more serious from of susto, though it is not to be confused with susto pasado or susto meco, which are even more serious because they have been permitted to persist. Nor is desasombro as serious as espanto, which will be discussed next. Desasombro should be thought of as a susto with a more significant cause. If stepping on a snake resulted in susto, stepping on a poisonous snake would result in desasombro.

Espanto

This, like susto, is a form of spirit loss, but it is much more severe. The difference between the two, as delineated by Dolores Latorre, will explain why this is so. Latorre writes that

> *susto* takes place when the victim is in possession of his spirit, and, although the spirit may temporarily leave the body due to the fright, the spirit is believed to be nearby and can easily be persuaded to return to the body through the prescribed ritual. *Espanto*, on the other hand, occurs when a person is asleep. Since at this time, the spirit may leave the body to wander far and wide during dreams, it may not be nearby to return into the body when entreated.

She goes on to outline the causes of espanto. These include being awakened suddenly by something frightening—say, a burglar or a disaster such as a fire or flood, by falling out of bed, or by a nightmare.

Bilis

This is best described as having excessive bile in the system. It is thought to be brought about by suppressed anger. Symptoms include gas, constipation, a pasty-looking tongue, and sour taste in the mouth.

Muína

This, Dolores Latorre reports, is sometimes called "anger sickness," but it differs from bilis in that it results from a show of rage rather than its suppression. The victim, Latorre writes, "becomes tied up in knots, trembles, and may lose the ability to talk or may become momentarily paralyzed. The jaws may lock, or hearing may stop." Like bilis, muína can result in a discharge of bile throughout the body. Latorre says that it can lead to jaundice.

Latido

Originally, the symptoms of latido, which translates as "palpitation" or "throb," were weakness, and a throbbing, jumpy feeling in the pit of the stomach. Now, however, the term latido is often used to describe a stomachache. Both forms of latido tend to strike those who are weak and thin.

Some liken latido to a nervous stomach, though others, probably describing the original ailment, say it is like the condition which medical authorities call hypoglycemia (low blood sugar). Indeed, symptoms of latido usually occur when a person has not eaten for a long period of time.

Envidia, mal puesto, salar, maleficio

These are all the result of evil-doing, and most are motivated by envy (or, less often, revenge). The threat of these ills is often enough to make a person live modestly, never making an obvious show of anything that might inspire the jealousy of another.

Some of these conditions can be brought about by an individual, but often the individual will engage the services of a witch, or brujo, sometimes called a black curandero. Most curanderos, however, are white curanderos—not those who cause illness, but rather those who heal in the name of God.

A curandero who is not a witch, fortunately, can remove a hex or spell. Or, as happens less frequently, a black curandero can be hired to counter it with a spell of his own. Indeed, sometimes feuds or battles between black curanderos have been recorded. Patrick Boulay, writing in the *San Antonio Light*, notes, for example, "Of nine curanderos The Light attempted to track down, three had died and one contracted a serious illness at the time the last battle was said to have occurred." One of the people Boulay interviewed for the article said that feuds between black curanderos "have taken a tremendous toll in San Antonio."

More often, a curandero who is not a witch (and most aren't) will be called upon to cure an ailment brought about by witchcraft. This is true even of the most famed curanderos.

In one story, a woman reported witnessing the seizure of still another woman who was *embrujada*—bewitched. The seizure took place in the presence of the famous Don Pedrito Jaramillo of Falfurrias, Texas. Don Pedrito, according to the account in Ruth Dodson's *The Healer of Los Olmos*, attempted without success to revive the woman, who had lost consciousness. The woman is said to have awakened, but during another seizure, long after leaving Don Pedrito's, she is rumored to have fallen into an open fire where she burned to death.

The famous curandero of Espinazo, Mexico, Niño Fidencio, is said to have left posterity a formula against being hexed. It requires, according to Dolores Latorre, that an aloe vera plant be tied with a red ribbon knotted twelve times and that a lime be attached to the plant with yet another red ribbon. Both should be looped around the aloe

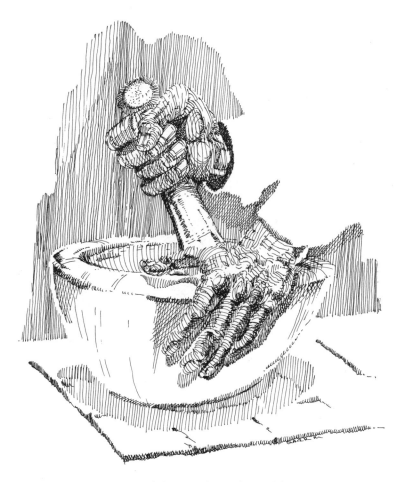

Figure 4: Many of the rituals performed by curanderos
include a mixture of several plants.

vera's roots and then the plant should be suspended, upside down, above the inside of the front door. But this alone was not enough! Each Friday before sunrise, the plant had to be taken outdoors and placed in water until just before noon. When the plant was brought inside again, the water in which it had soaked was to be sprinkled around the house. Whether this was an effective preventative or simply something to take one's mind off witchcraft and hexing is not known. These stories do demonstrate, however, that even the most famous of curanderos have had to deal with brujos and their work!

Chapter Four

The Rituals

While many of these ailments require that the patient eat, drink, or otherwise use a specific substance—such as an herb—their cure also involves ritual and the use of what an anthropologist would call "symbolic objects." To define the latter, think of the stereotypical view of the jungle "witch doctor" as presented in movies or even comic books: in all likelihood, he wears a mask and carries bones or a rattle. Well, the mask, the bones, and the rattle are clearly "symbolic objects." They are supposed to have a certain power in whatever ceremony the "witch doctor" performs.

A curandero uses symbolic objects, too, but because he feels his power comes from God, the symbols are those that are shared by many religious people who are not healers: the cross, pictures of saints, votive candles, and the like.

The curandero also uses everyday materials: olive oil, water, or, most commonly, an egg. The modern curandera, María, who was interviewed on KPRC-TV in Houston, said that she uses growing plants. "These plants . . . are very sensitive to their surroundings,"

María said. "When I tell a person that I am going to work on a particular problem for them . . . if they have an illness of some sort, then what I do is I tell them to buy me a plant. When they buy me a plant, they have automatically put their own vibrations . . . their own thoughts, feelings . . . negative and positive . . . into the plant. The reason a plant works is that, once a ritual has been performed, where the plant takes on the identity of that person, a spiritual link is formed between that plant and that person. No other person can take on the identity of the plant and vice versa."

Don Pedrito often used mere water, instructing patients to drink, for example, a glass at bedtime each night for a certain number of nights.

But the egg figures in most rituals of curanderismo, past and present. Earl Thompson, a novelist of astonishing talent, described one such ritual in *Caldo Largo*:

> (The curandera) straightened Lupe's body so she lay face up like a corpse, even crossing her hands on her breasts. As she crossed her hands, she slipped something into Lupe's palms, closed her hands into fists, and told her to hold what she had put in them very tight.
>
> "What is it?" Lupe asked.
>
> "Herbs. Now don't talk again until I tell you."
>
> The curandera placed candles on the table at Lupe's head and feet. She then poured some fragrant oil from a bottle that had once held tequila into her own large hands, warmed it between her palms and began to work it back through Lupe's hair until her thick reddish tresses were fanned around her face and down over her breasts and body until Lupe gleamed with the oil, all the while chanting some sort of prayer which I could not understand except for the occasional mention of the mother of Jesus. It was in a dialect I

had never beard before. It was hypnotic. I thought Lupe had gone to sleep or fallen into a trance. She seemed hardly to breathe. The smell of the oil was that of jasmine mixed with fresh herbs. The room was very warm and close . . .

She massaged Lupe front and back and front again, chanting all the while. The last time she had Lupe hold the egg in her clasped hands on her breast.

Then she took the egg from her and began gently rubbing it over her forehead, face, neck, and shoulders and then over the rest of her body. She traced the perimeters of Lupe with the egg as if drawing a pattern of her . . .

She then described a cross on her with the egg . . . she brought the egg to rest finally on Lupe's navel.

Compare the ritual undergone by Lupe to those described by Trotter and Chavira in their book on curanderismo, written to provide health care professionals with a better understanding of the subject. While rituals vary in detail from healer to healer, they have a common theme.

Mal ojo, the two say,

is treated by having the child lie down and sweeping him three times with an egg. The sweeping is done by forming crosses with the egg, on the child's body, starting at the head and going to the feet. While sweeping, the healer recites the Apostles' Creed three times, making sure that he sweeps both the front and the back. The egg is cracked and dropped into a glass or jar filled with water. The jar may then be placed on the child's head, and another Creed recited. The jar is then placed under the child's bed, usually under the place where the child rests his head. The next morning at sunrise the egg may either be burned or cast away in the form of a cross.

In a book intended for school children titled *Discovering Folklore Through Community Resources*, the ritual described to cure ojo is very similar, though less solemn in that, in the morning, the egg can either be buried or flushed down the toilet. The egg, once it is broken into the water, too, is used for diagnosis: "If the white becomes solid and forms an oval (an eye-shaped ring), people believe that the patient has indeed been suffering from a case of *ojo* and that he has been cured."

A curandero whom Ari Kiev interviewed said: "You have to break an egg and say a prayer. You break your egg, put it in the glass, and then put some little piece from the broom, you know, on top like a cross, and then the egg starts bubbling. You have to brush (the victim) with the egg first—make like a cross. The egg takes out the evil from the child and makes the person causing it stop ... When the egg starts boiling, that is when you know he had *ojo*. When the egg goes down, if it does not boil, it means that he doesn't have the *ojo*."

Remember the woman whom Evelyne Winter interviewed? When her husband was rubbed with the egg, first it was hard-boiled afterwards, then coddled, and finally raw. It was only when the egg emerged raw that the curandero considered the man cured.

The ritual for curing susto involves a broom. As Trotter and Chavira describe it:

> The sick person lies down and is completely covered with a sheet. The healer sweeps the patient with the broom, saying the Apostles' Creed three times. At the end of each Creed, the healer whispers in the patient's ear, "Come, don't stay there." The patient responds, "I am coming." The sick person must perspire and is then given some tea of *yerba anís* [aniseed] to drink. The healer then places a cross of holy palm on the patient's head and asks Almighty God, in the name of the Holy Trinity, to restore the patient's spiritual strength.

The cure for susto, which Dolores Latorre describes, involves both the broom and the egg:

> The cure must be done on three consecutive nights: Wednesday, Thursday, and Friday, the last day being the most effective. The patient lies on the bed with arms extended in the form of a cross while his entire body is cleansed with an alum rock or a whole egg and he is swept with a bundle or broom of herbs, preferably horehound, rosemary, California peppertree, redbrush, or naked-seed weed, tied together or separately. Each evening, fresh herbs are used.

Both rituals involve an invocation to the patient's spirit to return, and the patient's reply. In Trotter and Chavira, the appropriate response is said to be "*Aquí vengo*," while Latorre reports that "*Hay voy*" is used. Both may be interpreted as an affirmative response suggesting that the spirit is indeed returning.

Discovering Folklore Through Community Resources reports, as did Latorre, that the cure takes place over a Wednesday, Thursday, and Friday, but shows a curandera first blessing the susto victim's bed with a knife. The healer then sweeps the patient with *cenizo* (a sage-like plant) and blesses him with holy water. The Apostles' Creed is used in this ritual as well, but in addition to it, the curandera recites from her own personal prayer book. Only then does she call the spirit, enjoining it to return. After the ritual, the herbs used to sweep the patient are taken home to be placed under the patient's pillow in the form of a cross.

Ari Kiev describes sweeping, too, but the curanderos he interviewed suggested that *granada* (pomegranate) leaves be used. One of Kiev's healer informants reported that occasionally massage with an egg was also used for susto.

Don Pedrito, whose cures were often unconventional, is said to have cured a susto by divining what had caused it (the victim had witnessed a murder) and prescribing that a draught of beer be drunk on three successive nights. Still another legend about Don Pedrito is that he once cured one susto by subjecting the victim to another fright, in fact, appearing to the victim in the guise of a bandit to provide the scare! Both of these stories were gathered by Ruth Dodson in *The Healer of Los Olmos*.

The treatment for caída de mollera is more standard. As Kiev reports, "It involves turning the baby over on his heels, pushing up with the thumb against the roof of the child's mouth, packing the fontanelle area with moist salt, and/or binding the area."

"Binding" the area is smearing it with a sticky substance—either soap or egg white. It is not uncommon to see babies who have had this treatment out in public.

The thumb is usually used to push against the roof of the baby's mouth.

An egg can be used to pinpoint the site of the blockage causing empacho. A Mexican-American mother whom Kiev interviewed, for instance, tells of her method of diagnosis: "To treat it, you rub their stomach real good and rub them with an egg at room temperature, not from the fridge, and then you rub their stomach real good with it. Wherever that egg burst, that is where the *empacho* is in the stomach."

More often, a massage, followed by the administration of a laxative, is used. The same woman concludes the description of treatment thusly: "Then they tie a piece of linen around to hold it there. After they do all the rubbing and applying of the egg, they give them a good dose of castor oil or something to make them move their bowels."

Trotter and Chavira found this combination: "In some cases the healer massages that part of the back behind the stomach with warm olive oil and pulls on the skin. The skin is said to make a snapping noise when the trapped food particles are loosened. In either case, a tea is given to treat the damaged stomach."

One home remedy is to rub the patient's stomach with shortening and—again, this conveys the notion of loosening something that is stuck—pulling the skin on the patient's back until it pops.

Mal aire is treated like a cold—with tea, lemon juice, even whiskey. Liniments and poultices are used, too.

The treatment for desasombro is much more elaborate, for it is a much more serious ill. One popular curing method is outlined in *Discovering Folklore Through Community Resources*. The treatment is to be done outdoors at eleven in the morning. It begins when the curandero digs four holes in the ground in the shape of a diamond. One hole is for the head, one for the feet, and two are for the hands. The area is covered with a white sheet, and the patient stretches out, face down, in the form of a cross atop it, with his limbs in the appropriate spots. Another white sheet is placed atop him. The curandero, reciting the Apostles' Creed, then sweeps the patient from top to bottom.

It is interesting to note that in various recorded remedies for susto, curanderos have been quite specific about what should be used for the sweeping. In one case it was granada and in another cenizo, for instance. The ritual outlined above says that an ordinary household broom can be used.

This illustrates how these rituals are adapted according to what is available.

In any case, the curandero sweeps the patient and recites the Apostles' Creed three times as he does so. The patient rolls over, face up, hands still outstretched in the form of a cross. The sweeping ritual is repeated.

Now the patient is uncovered and stands. The curandero strikes the patient's shadow. Then the curandero drags a piece of clothing that the patient has worn into the patient's house, calling the spirit as he does so. He continues to call until he reaches the patient's bed. The patient comes in, sits on the bed, and drinks a cup of anís tea. The patient finishes drinking, leaving a bit of the tea in the cup.

Next the curandero takes some of the dirt that was removed from the four holes he dug when the ritual began. This dirt is mixed with the tea that the patient left. With the resulting mud, the curandero marks the sign of the cross on each of the patient's joints.

The patient then gets under as many covers as it will take to make him sweat. The curandero sweeps the patient now with cenizo and completes the ritual by reciting the Apostles' Creed three more times.

Treatment for bilis is far less exotic. Epsom salts or some other laxative would be given once each week for three weeks. On the other hand, the treatment for muína—the other illness caused by anger—is very formulaic. As Dolores Latorre reports: "The affected person is swept with three red flowers on three consecutive days, Wednesday, Thursday, and Friday, and afterward is given a decoction made with flowers and leaves of the orange tree or other citrus. This will calm the patient. If it does not, the person is struck, shaken, or addressed with unkind words in order to break the fit of anger." Interestingly, the symptoms that Latorre attributes to muína (given earlier in this book) are much like those of someone we would call hysterical. Even today, an hysterical person is slapped or shaken, much the way the victim of muína would be if he didn't respond to the ritual of the flowers.

Latido is usually treated by administering nourishment. Some suggest that a patient take, for nine consecutive days, a mixture of raw egg, salt, pepper, and lemon juice. A more appetizing cure requires that the patient eat bean soup with onion, coriander, and garlic. Latorre describes a *comfortativo* made of a hard roll called a bolillo, which is split, sprinkled with alcohol, and filled with peppermint leaves, nasturtiums, some cinnamon, cloves, and onions. After this is done, the roll is closed, wrapped in white cloth, and bandaged over the pit of the patient's stomach.

The fact is, as far-fetched as some of these rituals may sound to those of us accustomed to the cold, sterile administration of

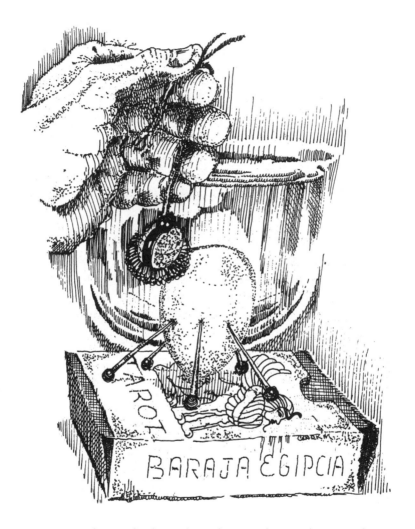

Figure 5: The seed-adorned amulet, ojo de venado, is used to ward off mal do ojo while the tarot cards are used by a señora to predict health, home life, and social conditions.

medical aid, they work! And as the story from Evelyne Winter's book demonstrated, one does not have to believe in the cures in order for them to work.

Perhaps most importantly, the curandero focuses his attention one hundred percent on his patient. This must be a significant component of the healing process.

Then, too, touch figures largely in the healing rituals. Only recently has the medical establishment come to acknowledge the therapeutic importance of touch.

The rituals often involve other members of the patient's family, too, and many are done in the patient's own home. The person who is ill thus has a very deep sense of belonging while the rituals are performed.

The status of the curandero also figures in his success. As Ari Kiev points out: "The curandero is never in doubt as to the diagnosis or treatment and does not undermine confidence in himself among nontechnically oriented patients by ordering laboratory tests and X-rays. He turns to meaningful sources of strength such as the saints and God."

Chapter Five

Folk Beliefs

There are numerous beliefs associated with curanderismo that do not necessarily have to do with illness. Many of these involve the color red. A red thread laid across the forehead of a person with hiccups is said to cure them. A red ribbon, tied in knots to represent the problems of a person, when buried, is said to rid that person of the problems the knots represent. A red dress, worn by a mother, is rumored to cure an apathetic or listless child.

Red is considered the color of love, and it figures in love-related ceremonies. A San Antonio curandera melted two red candles together, molding them by hand into something resembling the human form, in order to reunite a separated couple. In the same ritual, water tinted red was also used.

There are many beliefs involving preventatives. The ojo de venado or deer's eye charm, which keeps its wearer safe from mal de ojo, is one. A bag of parsley worn about the neck is said to ward off snakes. A pregnant woman is advised to hang some keys around her waist during a lunar eclipse to keep her baby from being deformed by the moon's shadow.

Beliefs about the moon itself are interesting. It is thought, for instance, that a person can become bewitched by the moon—*alunado*.

Simply carrying a bud of garlic (*ajo macho*) is supposed to protect against a host of potential ills.

A *barrida* or spiritual cleansing is a preventative ritual performed by a curandero. It serves to eliminate negative influences by transferring them to another object. Trotter and Chavira describe the ceremony:

> Patients are swept from their head to their feet, with the curandero making sweeping or brushing motions with an egg, a lemon, an herb, or whatever appropriate object is deemed necessary. According to some informants the object must be held in the curandero's left hand and must touch the person being swept. . . . Standard prayers used in this ritual include the Lord's Prayer, the Apostles' Creed . . .

An article in the *San Antonio Light* mentioned several preventatives—mainly amulets or, in Spanish, *amuletos*:

> Many are made of what looks like dirt, glitter, gold colored corn, a broken cross-shaped twig painted silver with metal shavings packaged in a cellophane bag.
>
> Candles are also a common item. They come in various colors, each denoting a particular meaning.
>
> Burning a black candle brings freedom from evil, a blue candle brings peace, harmony and joy, and a red candle denotes love and affection.

An old wife's tale reminds pregnant women to burn pink colored incense and look at a colored picture of St. Ramón. This is supposed to be good for the mother and her unborn child.

Another long-term practice is the idea of putting a coin in the mouth of the image of St. Ramón so bad things won't be said about you.

Proponents of curanderismo have enormously strong beliefs in luck and do what they can to court it. Various types of incense are used for this purpose. Not only was incense used in Aztec and Mayan ceremonies, but it figured largely in the Judeo-Christian past as well. The three wise men, or Magi, for example, were said to bring the Christ child gifts of gold, frankincense, and myrrh. And, of course, in Roman Catholic celebrations—either in the Mass or at a Benediction, to name two such events—incense was often used. Today, in Mexican and Mexican-American herb shops (*yerberias*), one can find the traditional incense that is burned as well as various aerosol varieties.

Michael Quintanilla, in the *San Antonio Express-News*, catalogued a good many offerings in one typical urban Mexican-American *botica,* or drugstore: "Each vial has a purpose and no two are alike. The various vials claim to bring the wearer good luck, more money, success or movie-star good looks in addition to Cupid's arrow. They can also work to ward off the jealousy and envy of others or those who want to see the wearer fail in life, marriage or business."

Perfumes and oils, too, are popular. Quintanilla quotes the owner of the store: "For wealth, he says, a dab or two of *Exito* (Success) will have the wearer rolling in dough . . . And, if all else fails, *Una Gota de Suerte* (One Drop of Luck) is bound to be the definitive fire water to solving your agony, ridding your hex, curing your illness, or getting

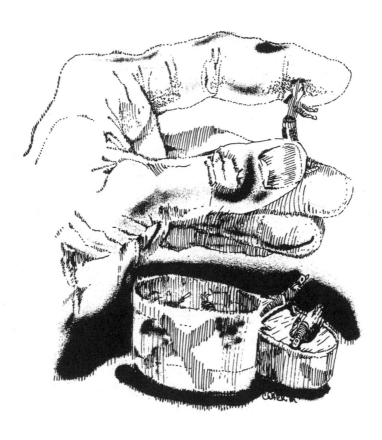

Figure 6: One's worries are transferred to six trouble dolls, each representing a particular problem.

back at someone. Like an all-purpose cleaner, *Una Gota* will clean up the mess in your life."

An Austin freelance writer, now living in New York, says that she went on assignment to a place in Houston known to sell the items used in curanderismo. She jokingly told the woman behind the counter that she needed something to change her life. The woman returned with something called Special Brown Oil.

"It smelled like the kind of disinfectant they use in public rest rooms." The writer laughs, but she dutifully dabbed it on as she'd been directed. "The next week," the writer says, "I had a call from a publishing company. They wanted to publish my doctoral dissertation, which I'd done more than ten years earlier. Then an old boyfriend called—my high school sweetheart." The writer is now engaged to marry him. "Trouble is," she says, only half joking, "I'm almost out of the oil!"

Questions about the sort of luck the future will bring are common. Trotter and Chavira report that every curandero to whom they spoke had knowledge of card readers, or señoras, who have a particular specialty. These use either the tarot, the fifty-two card American deck, or the forty card Mexican deck. "These *señoras* make specific predictions," the authors say, "normally in three areas: health, home life, and social condition (including legal and business matters)."

Perhaps the most interesting thing about Mexican-American folk medicine is that its believers rely upon, transfer to, or blame — to a remarkable degree—objects and causes that are external. Nowhere is this more obvious than in the use of what are called Trouble Dolls—recently quite popular.

These small figures reside in a gaily-decorated box. At night, the troubled person removes a number of dolls—one to represent each of his problems. The dolls are then placed back inside the box. In the morning, the dolls will have assumed all of the person's woes! This is said to work very well with children.

Chapter Six

Don Pedrito Jaramillo

W hen author James Michener was researching his book on Texas, one of the first things he did was visit the burial site of Don Pedrito Jaramillo. Most historians would agree that Don Pedrito is the most famous curandero of all time. In fact, some seventy-five years after Don Pedrito's death, *Texas Monthly* magazine called him "one of the most powerful men in South Texas."

The *Texas Monthly* article (January 1982) was titled "The Saint of Falfurrias," and indeed, that is what Don Pedrito has become: a folk saint—a personage to whom people pray in order to combat their illness, change their luck or their habits, or as an expression of their faith.

In 1964, Octavio Romano, a doctoral candidate in Anthropology at the University of California at Berkeley, did his dissertation on the phenomenon. It was called "Don Pedrito Jaramillo: The Emergence of a Mexican-American Folk-Saint." A folk saint, as Romano defines it, is "a deceased person who is considered a saint by the people but not by the Catholic Church." This, he says, is "relatively rare."

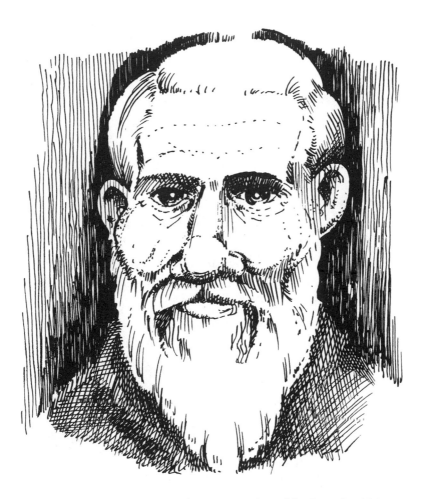

Figure 7: Don Pedrito used water, mud, and herbs to heal his clients. His tombstone reads "The Benefactor of Humanity."

A visitor to the shrine of Don Pedrito might be disappointed to find it is a simple, tin-roofed shed. Inside, however, are a myriad of candles lit in gratitude or in petition. There are crutches affixed to the wall and tucked beneath the beams of the ceiling. And everywhere there are drawings, handmade thank-you cards, and other items left behind to link the believer with the healer. Drivers' licenses, because they carry the believer's photograph, are thought to be especially potent when asking Don Pedrito for help. In truth, very little of the original wall space at the Falfurrias shrine can be seen because of these items.

And, of course, at almost any hour of the day, someone will be there, kneeling in prayer.

The land upon which the shrine is built was known, in Don Pedrito's lifetime, as *Los Olmos*—The Elms. There were occasions when the surrounding countryside was thronged with those seeking the healer's aid. In addition, each mail delivery brought hundreds of petitions from those unable to make the trip in person. At one point, postal authorities suspected Don Pedrito of some sort of fraud, because the outgoing replies were far in excess of the number expected, using the stamps sold at the small rural post office as a guide. The postal investigators were appeased when they learned that most of the people who wrote enclosed stamps to insure a reply.

The definitive biographical details come from Ruth Dodson, who collected lore about Don Pedrito over a great many years and who published it, first in Spanish and later in English, as *The Healer of Los Olmos*, under the sponsorship of Southern Methodist University and the Texas Folklore Society. What follows is a condensed version of Don Pedrito Jaramillo's life and miracles.

Don Pedrito's given name was Pedro Jaramillo and this is what his tombstone reads. Pedrito is a diminutive of Pedro, and Don is a title of respect. Interestingly, curanderos often refer to their ability to heal as a don, which means "gift" in Spanish.

Don Pedrito was born in 1829 in Mexico. Nothing is known of his childhood, but he was either a shepherd or a laborer; in any case, he was poor.

Don Pedrito is said to have asked God to heal his mother, pledging that, if his mother were not healed, he would leave Mexico. Thus, when his mother died, Don Pedrito crossed the border into Texas.

This was 1881, which would make him fifty-two years old when he came to Falfurrias. Another item of note is that Don Pedrito is said to have known the area, having once come that way to deliver alcoholic beverages to one of the ranches there.

Don Pedrito is said to have learned of his healing gift when he suffered a fall from a horse (even later in his life, he was said to have been, at best, a mediocre horseman). In the fall, he injured his nose. In the days that followed, the pain was excruciating. Then something led him to a nearby wallow where he, for no reason he could name, dabbed mud all over the injured spot. This assuaged the pain and he was able to sleep. During that sleep, Don Pedrito said that God spoke to him, telling him to spend the rest of his life healing the sick and injured. From that day forward, this is what Don Pedrito did.

Many of his cures, like the one that he applied to himself, involved bathing. Mud—earth and water—did not cost his patients a cent. Other of his cures involved a simple ritual: drinking a glass of water, for instance, for a prescribed number of days—usually three or nine, the so-called mystical numbers.

It is said that, in addition to his ability to heal, Don Pedrito had psychic powers. Many of the legends about him note his uncanny ability to detect the unbelievers. Still other stories demonstrate that he could "read minds." On more than one occasion, particularly when someone who had suffered a susto came to him, he was able to pinpoint the traumatic event the person had undergone.

Some of the tales reveal Don Pedrito's sense of humor. One involves a woman with migraine headaches who sent a surrogate to seek a cure. The remedy that Don Pedrito prescribed was this: that the woman cut her head off and feed it to the hogs. The woman was so angry when the substitute she had sent came home and told her this that she sputtered and fumed—and never suffered another headache as long as she lived!

There are patients of Don Pedrito's who were reluctant to tell of the cures he had prescribed. There are others who reported that he asked his patients to do what seemed bizarre: one woman was to dip her head in a bucket of water before retiring, and then, in the morning, put half a can of tomatoes into each shoe! Indeed, there are even cures requiring that his patients consume large amounts of alcohol!

The thread common to all—and perhaps it is most visible in those cures that seem especially odd—is that the faith of the supplicant was thus tested. Some experts feel, then, that the very belief played a large role in the healing.

Surely this is true even in formal medicine. But what would those experts conclude in some of the cases involving animals? For instance, Dodson reports this cure: "A man had a very fine horse that got sick. Don Pedrito told the man to tie the horse to a chinaberry tree at twelve o'clock sharp, and at one o'clock sharp to take him away from the tree. With this the horse would get well and the chinaberry tree would die."

This is said to have worked!

One story that I especially like is about a man who drank water so quickly he had failed to notice a grass burr in it. This, he swallowed, and it stuck on the way down. A medical doctor told him only an operation could remove it, and so the man continued to suffer until he went to Don Pedrito. Don Pedrito's remedy was, as were all the things that he prescribed, utterly simple: the man should drink all the saltwater that he could. The man did so, became nauseated, and vomited up the burr, which—the story says—had by this time sprouted two little leaves.

Although many of these stories seem like they were written to amuse us, they are documented and presumably true accounts.

Don Pedrito, like other curanderos, did not take money for his services. What he did accept, he used to feed the pilgrims who came to Los Olmos, and to finance his travels to heal those who could not make the trip.

During a drought that struck South Texas in 1893 and lasted for many years, Don Pedrito is said to have fed enormous numbers of people. When the state of Texas sent food, Don Pedrito was selected to distribute it.

Rumor holds that someone he cured gave Don Pedrito his own son in gratitude. This has never been substantiated, but Don Pedrito, who never married and who never sired a son of his own, did adopt Severiano Barrera, who is now considered his descendant.

Don Pedrito died in 1907. His tombstone calls him "The Benefactor of Humanity," which, indeed, he was. He had asked that his grave be opened after three days, but, inexplicably, this was not done.

Chapter Seven

Niño Fidencio

Niño Fidencio's healing powers might not have come to the attention of all of Mexico had he not cured the daughter of Plutarco Elias Calles, then the president of that country. From that time forth, El Niño's fame—though he never ventured out of the small and dusty town of Espinazo—was assured.

Niño Fidencio had been born in Guanajuato. He came to Espinazo in 1925 at the bidding of a friend. It is said he was a sort of tutor, but, in legend anyway, he had been performing cures since the age of eight!

El Niño was born in 1898. He was forty when he died in 1938. Nonetheless, stories persist that he was thirty-three at his death—one of many conscious efforts to link Fidencio's life with the life of Jesus Christ of Nazareth.

El Niño had, for example, twelve disciples. He would often go to a nearby mountain to meditate—something that compares, some say, to Christ in the Garden of Gethsemane. In any case, this sort of parallel is very often drawn.

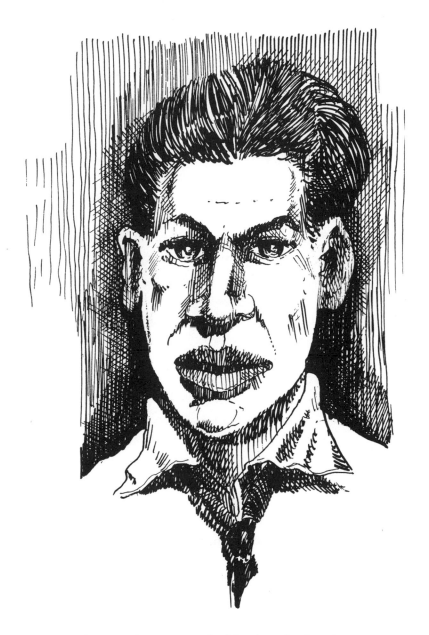

Figure 8: El Niño Fidencio prescribed laughter, food, and merriment, and his healings are still practiced by his followers called Fidencistas.

Niño Fidencio is remembered as a childlike, happy man. Indeed, for the hoards of sick and injured who came to him, he often prescribed laughter, food, and merriment. When anyone gave him gifts—and the President of Mexico seemed to do so with great frequency—El Niño used the occasion to share, thus lightening the otherwise gloomy existence of many of the pilgrims. There are stories that say that El Niño Fidencio hired musicians so that everyone—even arthritics and cripples—might dance. The same stories swear that everyone did just that!

Just as with Don Pedrito Jaramillo, there are humorous accounts of some of El Niño's cures. For instance, he is said to have cured a mute by making him stand in front of a swing. El Niño rocked in the swing and bumped into the man often enough to make him angry. The man, furious, found the voice that had eluded him for several years. Similarly, El Niño is said to have tricked a paralytic into standing by tossing sweets just out of her range had she continued to sit.

But there are other cures, too—cures sufficient to inspire some thirty thousand or more to trek to Espinazo twice a year (in March and in October, the anniversaries of his birth and death) to pay homage to the famous curandero. And those who come do so from all over the United States and Mexico. Some come year after year. Usually they are those who come in gratitude for a miraculous response to their prayers.

There is something special, however—something quite particular—about the way El Niño, as opposed to other curanderos, is praised, beseeched, or honored.

Those who are his followers—the *Fidencistas* who dress in white shirts and red kerchiefs—are said to assume his very spirit. They are called *cajones* (male) and *materias* (female) and act as *cajitas* (little boxes). They are thought, for the duration of their trance, to actually become El Niño.

Indeed, this has been observed by sociologists, who often make the pilgrimage as well. It is said that the most striking difference in those assuming El Niño's spirit is a softening—for El Niño is said to have been very gentle, very benign. The number of Fidencistas continues to grow, and there are shrines to Niño Fidencio, as mentioned in the introduction to this book, even in Northern cities throughout the United States.

Not everyone who goes to Espinazo is a Fidencista capable of this psychic feat. Most are simple folk whom El Niño has cured, or those who are hoping for a cure. In Espinazo, proofs of some of Niño Fidencio's cures abound, too. At his tomb, for instance, there are tumors he is said to have removed on display in formaldehyde-filled jars.

The people who wish to petition him arrive by car, on foot, or by rail to throng the narrow, unpaved streets. The first thing that they do, however, is circle the Pirul tree at the base of the hill three times. El Niño often sat under this tree. It has been named *El Pirulito* and has even been assigned its own caretaker!

Next, the people walk uphill to El Niño's burial site.

The road they walk is *El Camino de Penitencia* or The Road of Penance, and many of them interpret that literally, crawling, or walking on their knees the whole way.

Some locales choose to honor El Niño by sending not just a few folk, but a *misión,* a contingent of followers often costumed and bearing musical instruments. These go uphill in a more festive fashion than do those seeking to atone. Other groups, however, mirror the crucifixion of Christ, carrying long wooden crosses up the steep and dusty road.

Many choose to climb into a muddy trough at the top of the hill. It is here, at *El Charquito*, that El Niño is said to have bathed lepers.

Elsewhere throughout the town is a carnival-like atmosphere.

There are stalls with all sorts of native food as well as remembrances of the pilgrimage and El Niño for sale. There are medals bearing his image alongside those of established saints who are recognized by the Catholic Church. It is this that leads many to call El Niño, as they call Don Pedrito, a "folk saint." One very unusual religious image that appears rather often is Niño Fidencio's face superimposed upon the face of Our Lady of Guadalupe.

To be sure, Niño Fidencio is the most revered faith healer in the history of Mexico. He is often called "the curandero of curanderos." His believers paint a striking visual image of the man, who walked barefoot, wore a white tunic, and is said to have cured madmen as well as those with more conventional ills.

His death is shrouded in rumor and mystery. Some say his throat was slit while he was in a trance; others say that he died of exhaustion. The latter makes some sense as El Niño is said to have slept but three hours each night, so busy was he healing those in need. He also fasted regularly. When he did eat, he preferred fruits and vegetables to meat.

But biographical details of El Niño's life are not easy to come by. Most have been changed a bit, to enhance the legend. Citing the age of his death as thirty-three, for instance, is but one example.

But on one point all of the stories agree: that Niño Fidencio tirelessly dedicated himself to others.

Chapter Eight

Teresita

The life of Teresa Urrea, as documented by William Curry Holden, who researched the subject for some twenty years, reads like a movie script. Hers can be presented here more fully than the lives of the other curanderos precisely because of Holden's fine research.

Teresita was born in Mexico in 1873, the illegitimate daughter of a fourteen-year-old Indian peasant girl and a dashing but philandering member of the aristocracy. She lived for a while in a dirt-floored village hut, but evidently hankered after something more. Legend says she confronted her father demanding her rightful place, but she said in an interview that her father sent for her when she was sixteen years old.

Her father, Don Tomás Urrea, on this and other occasions, was evidently impressed by the girl's spirit. She did indeed go to live with him at *La Casa Grande*. He acknowledged her as his daughter forevermore.

The family lived on an enormous ranch at Cabora, and Teresita quickly apprenticed herself in an informal way to Huila, the woman

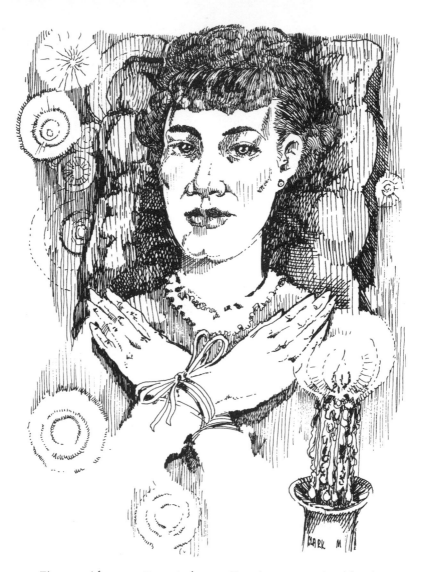

Figure 9: After an attempted rape, Teresita, traumatized by the experience, went into a coma and was thought to be dead. She was dressed for burial, her hands were bound across her breast, and candles were lit. But suddenly she sat upright, very much alive. Her powers were said to include hypnosis and prophecy, and she also prescribed herbs as part of the treatments she administered.

who distributed herbs and mended bones. Soon the old curandera realized that Teresita had powers that exceeded her own.

Hypnosis appeared to be one of them. On two occasions, Teresita, assisting Huila, was able to calm patients and, indeed, relieve them of their pain with her eyes alone. Huila is said to have reported her charge's gift to Don Tomás.

Prophecy was another of Teresita's powers. The first reported episode occurred when she was riding with a friend, Apolonaria. The two girls—then about sixteen years old—passed a dashing young stranger. Teresita startled Apolonaria by saying she had just met her future husband. What is more, she predicted Apolonaria's wedding day, more than two years hence!

A man who became enamored of Teresita attempted to rape her after she rebuffed him. Teresita was traumatized by the attack and began to have seizures. One resulted in a coma and, indeed, it seemed that Teresita had withdrawn into death.

She was dressed for burial, and her hands were bound across her breasts. Candles were lit. A coffin was built. The mourners gathered.

But suddenly Teresita sat upright, puzzled by the funeral preparations.

Three days later, however, Huila died. She was buried in the coffin that had been built for her beloved Teresita.

Teresita, from that day forth, assumed Huila's role as healer. In addition to preparing herbs and setting bones, however, she added her own aforementioned psychic feats.

Teresita's reputation grew, and soon La Casa Grande was over-run with those seeking her aid. Some of the occasions that were documented are dramatic indeed.

One man, carrying his paralyzed wife, was astounded to hear his name. "Fortunato Avendano, bring your wife to me," the voice called. Then it demanded that a way be cleared for the man. It was

Teresita's voice, of course, and she claimed to have known the pair would come.

After Teresita enabled Mariana, the wife, to walk—most say through a combination of hypnosis and massage—the couple pledged undying devotion. Indeed, they remained from that day forward in Teresita's employ.

But the hoards of people tramping through Cabora, most of whom needed to be fed, enraged Don Tomás. After one particularly weighty confrontation with his daughter, he is said to have come into her bedroom with a gun. He found he could not shoot, and from then on he did not argue.

Instead, he built separate quarters for his daughter, so that she could hold audiences with her followers without disturbing him or his holdings.

Not too long afterward, a reporter went to Cabora. His description of Teresita was:

Loveliness rather than beauty. What she has transcends beauty. It is something that projects. Projects and disarms . . . a warmth, a glow, eagerness and sincerity, a magnetism. Eyes that inspire confidence and faith, that probe and hypnotize. An arresting and remarkable woman. With the unconscious talent of a great actress, she establishes a spellbinding rapport with her audience. It is clear why believers find her irresistible. She tells them to walk and they walk. But for all her saintliness and good works, she is still a woman . . .

The reporter was soon to witness the first of many incidents that would lead him to believe with the others in Teresita's powers.

Meanwhile, under the dictatorship of Porfirio Díaz, Mexico, as Holden puts it, "became the safest place on earth for everyone except the unfortunate Mexicans and Indians."

Díaz made an agreement with the Roman Catholic Church in exchange for its support wherein he would not confiscate church property to reward his men. This meant the communal holdings of the Indians would be taken instead.

Teresita was a favorite among the Yaquis, who saw her as an oracle and who came to Cabora in great numbers. The Yaquis told her about Díaz's policy of confiscating their lands and asked for her advice. She told them, as she was later to tell the Mayo (not Mayan, who are a wholly different tribe) Indians who sought her counsel, to be patient and tolerant.

The *Mestizos* who inhabited Tomochic became devoted to her, too. In fact their leader, Cruz Chávez, began a lengthy correspondence with Teresita. But Chávez's devotion to Teresita went too far. Images of Teresita, for instance, were placed within the Tomochic church and the people prayed to these. Indeed, Chávez wrote an entire liturgy to accommodate the "living saint."

This was enough to inflame a Catholic priest, Father Manuel Gustelúm, to speak out against her from the Tomochic pulpit. The priest was stunned to hear himself contradicted immediately following his denouncement by none other than Cruz Chávez. The priest immediately reported the people of Tomochic to the government, saying they were in a state of rebellion.

This same priest had once crudely ordered that Teresita in her trance state be tested. What he had done was approach two nuns, extracting a hat pin from the headpiece of one, and asking that she use it to pierce the flesh of Teresita's leg. If she were indeed in a trance, the priest reasoned, she would not be injured, and if not, the fraud would be exposed. Under orders, the nuns went to Teresita's bedside and did what the priest had described. The pin went in one side of Teresita's calf and out the other without bleeding and, evidently, without inflicting pain since Teresita didn't stir from her trance state.

When she finally awakened of her own accord, she plucked the pin from her leg as if it were a minor irritant and told them to take it back to their priest.

It was this priest, then, who now had denounced the villagers who so idolized "La Santa de Cabora," their living saint.

Meanwhile, two other events had taken place. One occurred when the governor of the state of Chihuahua sent an envoy to remove two paintings—probably by Murillo—from the little village and hang, in their stead, two mediocre paintings. The men of Tomochic, led by Cruz Chávez, stopped the envoy and delivered a message to the governor on honesty.

This did not predispose the governor to ignore Father Gustelúm's claim now.

Simultaneously with Gustelúm's complaint came word that a caravan of expensive merchandise had gone around Tomochic for safety reasons.

When President Porfirio Díaz heard all of this, he was quick to conclude that the men of Tomochic were indeed revolting. He sent troops.

Cruz Chávez and his men heard this and went to Cabora to consult Teresita. When Díaz learned this, he ordered Chávez and his men apprehended, and Teresita placed under surveillance.

Government troops, led by a Captain Enrique, stormed Cabora. But Enrique was a friend of Don Tomás. The two men spoke, and Enrique told Don Tomás he had orders to arrest Teresita. Don Tomás and his sons swore they would give their lives in her defense. Enrique said he would withdraw his men while Don Tomás thought this over, and did so, giving Don Tomás and his daughter a chance to escape.

They rode to a government enclave and gave themselves up to a general whom, Don Tomás felt, would proffer justice.

Meanwhile, at Cabora, Enrique went in search of the approaching Cruz Chávez band, only to be slaughtered by them.

The general to whom Don Tomás and Teresita had turned themselves in ushered them back to Cabora, but, learning of Enrique's death, amassed several hundred men to quash Cruz Chávez.

Meanwhile, more events occurred to convince Díaz that Teresita was behind a movement toward revolution. Mayo Indians, for example, attacked a place called Navojoa convinced that "La Santa de Cabora" would protect them. These attacks included chants to the living saint. When Mayos began converging on Cabora, the government became convinced that Teresita—who was then but nineteen years old!—was directing the revolt.

In fact, there is some humor in the scene. A contingent of five hundred soldiers got to Cabora before the rumored influx of Mayos. Five hundred armed men confronting a nineteen-year-old girl!

But Díaz was not amused. He called Teresita a dangerous agitator and ordered her exiled. Thus she and her father were transported, under guard, to Nogales, Arizona.

Teresita's beauty was such that the commander in charge of escorting her out of the country left his horse to a friend and took the carriage seat beside his charge. He proposed marriage, then, rebuffed, suggested that they have a mere liaison. Teresita told Don Tomás, who threatened the man. This soldier did not complete the journey, but entrusted the transport to his next in command!

Arizona welcomed Teresita and she began curing a hundred patients a day.

Meanwhile, the Mexican government decided it had lost control of her movements by sending her out of the country. They wanted Teresita back.

After two kidnap attempts were made, Don Tomás moved with Teresita away from the Mexican border and into the interior of Arizona.

In Mexico, Cruz Chávez was still honoring Teresita, and, indeed, was fighting the federal soldiers under a banner made by the Tomochic women bearing the legend "La Santa de Cabora." The government brutally slaughtered Cruz Chávez and every male over the age of thirteen at Tomochic. President Díaz blamed the need for this hideous government action on Teresita.

In Arizona, a pro-revolution newspaper editor who had been exiled with Teresita and her father tried unsuccessfully to have Teresita endorse his cause. He decided to link her to his movement anyway, thus further convincing Díaz of her guilt. What he did was print a photograph of Teresita with her name and the words *La Espíritu de Tomochic* beneath it.

Her enemies needed little more, but more was to follow nonetheless. Though Teresita moved to El Paso and was healing two hundred patients a day, bands of revolutionaries continued to attack the government of Mexico in her name. In one organized attack from New Mexico, Arizona, and Texas, the rebels called themselves *Teresistas*. And most who were killed were found to be wearing the photograph captioned without her knowledge over their hearts.

Attempts were made on Teresita's life, either by agents of the government of Mexico or the fanatic followers of Father Gustelúm. Don Tomás had her moved to Clifton, Arizona.

This was, evidently, an idyllic time. Visitors came from as far away as Mexico City and New York City. Patients, however, were few. Thus Teresita resumed her old gaiety, playing the marimbas and guitar, and singing.

In 1899, at the age of twenty-seven, she fell in love.

An odd version of the shotgun wedding ensued. Don Tomás refused Guadalupe Rodriguez Teresita's hand, and Lupe, as he was called, hoisted a carbine and demanded it! Teresita went to Lupe's side and did marry him, though the marriage was never consummated.

The couple spent the entire night at a party, and the following day, Lupe told Teresita to follow him, though he stayed far ahead. She did follow, and he turned, pulled a gun, and tried to shoot her—something she had predicted years earlier.

Lupe was jailed and judged insane, though later it was suspected that he was in the employ of Díaz, hired either to lure Teresita back to Mexico or prove that she was dead.

Meanwhile, so much of a rift had occurred between Don Tomás and Teresita over her marriage that she thought it best to leave. She went to California, ostensibly to cure the child of a relative. She was never to see her father again.

In San Francisco, Teresita's cures amazed the populace and brought her large-scale publicity. In the wake of this, a medical company signed her to a contract and sent her on tour. In St. Louis, she found her lack of English handicapped her, and sent a plea for assistance to a friend back home.

The friend's bilingual son, John Van Order, then nineteen, joined Teresita in St. Louis to act as interpreter. Soon word came to Arizona that the pair were "married"—impossible since, legally, Teresita was the wife of Lupe. Interestingly, when descendants or others who had known Teresita were asked about her sainthood, they always disputed it, claiming she had been married. As author William Curry Holden points out, virginity was not demanded of male saints!

In any case, during this period, Teresita and John lived in an apartment in New York City (110 East 28th Street). In 1902, their daughter, Laura, was born. That same year, Teresita learned of the death of Don Tomás.

Though John and Teresita seemed less close with each passing day, in 1904, they had another child, a girl again. Christened Magdalena, the child was born in Clifton, Arizona, where Teresita, no longer touring for the medical company, had returned.

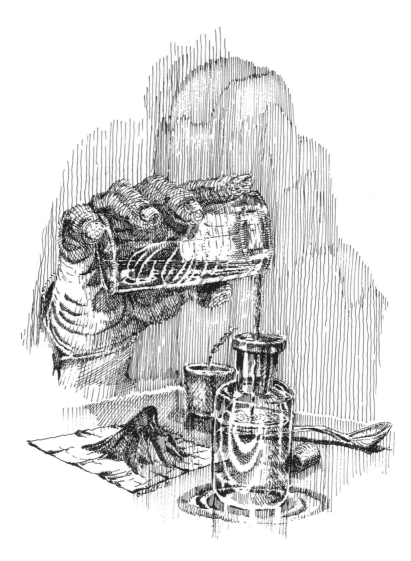

Figure 10: In addition to performing healing rituals, curanderos prescribe herbs in various forms—as fresh and dried plants, and sometimes in oils, tinctures, and liniments.

She seemed reduced, diminished. Her healing powers no longer seemed spectacular, and she, herself, was weak. She developed "lung trouble," and even had to stop seeing patients because of its contagion.

Before she died, she sought out her long lost mother, Cayetana, the Indian peasant who had bourn her at the age of fourteen. This reunion occurred just days before Teresita's death in 1906. She was buried in Clifton next to Don Tomás.

Chapter Nine

Modern Curanderos

This book has emphasized the rituals of curanderismo and the folk ailments they can cure. It should not be forgotten, however, that this is a distorted emphasis. Curanderos can, and usually do, treat organic ailments such as migraine, flu, even cancer. In fact, many of the folk ailments mentioned here can be treated by a family member. It is common to call in a curandero if the ailment persists or if it is a particularly severe case.

It is by virtue of this that an *El Proyecto Comprender* script is able to refer to the practice of curanderismo as "an optional health care system." The description of the curandero, as it appears there, is worth quoting, summarizing, as it does, the reasons for the marked efficacy of curanderismo:

> The strength of the curandero's success lies in the establishment of a personal relationship with his patient. He shares with his patient the same culture, language, and many of the same health beliefs and practices. Many Mexican-American

families have a long-standing relation with one particular curandero, much the same as they might have with a family physician. A curandero may be compared to a small town physician: he serves a relatively small number of patients, he knows the families intimately, and therefore is well-prepared to treat his patient's physical, psychological, and spiritual needs.

And, as Professor Robert Trotter from Pan American University pointed out in an interview with the *Corpus Christi Caller Times*, the modern curandero is not by any means uncivilized or barbaric. "People try to make curanderos different," Trotter says. "They equate them with what can be found in New Guinea. But curanderos are a part of an urban, industrialized society. They watch television, they know about Anacin and Bufferin and the modern health care system. They're not primitive."

Still, even a factual and pro-curanderismo article, quoted out of context, can make the practices sound very peculiar indeed. The following is from Jennifer Bloch, writing in the *Dallas Times Herald*:

[W]ithout a thought for the professors and physicians who write them off as superstitious, these simple, humble men and women go right on lighting candles, saying prayers, sweeping people with eggs and incense and lemons, anointing them with specially prepared oils and waters, brewing up herb teas, invoking spirits. Healing. Healing bodies, minds and spirits, tummy aches and terrors.

In capsule form, the practice of curanderismo cannot be adequately portrayed.

Robert Trotter is wise to enjoin us not to forget that the contemporary curandero is no stranger to the so-called miracle drugs and methods of modern science. "In Mexico," Trotter says, "curanderos prescribe antibiotics as well as *te de manzanilla* (chamomile tea) because such medicine is sold across the counter there without a necessary doctor's prescription. Here in the United States, the curanderos are restricted with what they can tell the patient to take. They know the value of penicillin, so they also know when it's time to refer their patients to a medical doctor."

Methods differ; time alters some practices (for example, aerosol sprays are sometimes substituted for incense). On the other hand, consider the striking similarity between Teresita's mode of healing as she explained it in a 1900 *San Francisco Examiner* interview with Helen Dare, and that of a modern curandero or, for that matter, a contemporary holistic practitioner:

> "When I cure with my hands I do like this," and she took my hands in hers—hands of singular slenderness and fineness, cool, smooth, supple, firm, delicately made, charming to touch—and placed her thumbs against mine, holding with a close nervous grasp.
>
> "Sometimes," she said, "I rub, sometimes I give also medicines or lotions that I make from herbs I gather. I pray, too, not with the lips, but I lift up my spirit to God for help to do His will on earth."

That Teresita's method would be soothing cannot be denied. One can almost feel her touch, hear her voice, as one reads! Conversely, Don Pedrito would give prescriptions or *recetas*—a method much more similar to contemporary medical practice. One such prescription—and it can be considered typical—was: "Don Feliciano, in the name of God, your wife and your mother should each take a cup of cold water for seven nights at bedtime."

Most of Don Pedrito's cures were transmitted this way, perhaps because so many of his clients approached him through messengers or by using the mail.

Is curanderismo legal? In Mexico, of course, there is no problem, and this is why in border towns, where patients can cross the border at will, curanderismo is so strong. Even a famous healer like Don Pedrito, however, had difficulties with the law. This occurred in San Antonio, where Don Pedrito drew quite a crowd and therefore the attention of police. When they found he charged nothing for his services, they stopped harassing him.

Most curanderos can work openly and freely today. An article in the *San Antonio Light* explains, "In Texas, curanderos operate with the tacit approval of the Catholic Church, whose religious symbolism the healers often appropriate, and of the State Board of Medical Examiners. (The board focuses on licensing doctors and investigating complaints against individual MDs and other providers of health care. So far, no complaints have been filed against curanderos.)" This observation by reporters Patrick Boulay and Allan Turner was made in 1981.

Just as Teresita and Don Pedrito—both curing during roughly the same time period—were markedly different, so are curanderos today. A television presentation by KPRC-TV News in Houston made this very clear. María, for example, a young curandera mentioned earlier in this book, wore no special garb. She used, if you remember, plants to absorb the patient's negative forces. And, contradicting what is usually the case, María charged a set fee. Her male counterpart on the television program, however, was a man perhaps in his sixties. He wore satin robes and a peaked satin cap of the sort one might associate with wizardry. He used a sword, too, and threatened the evil from the body of the woman who had come to him as a patient.

Not surprisingly, the patient with whom he was shown was an older woman. Again, not surprisingly, many of María's patients were young professionals, and a number were Anglo—that is, not Mexican-Americans.

There are even Anglo healers who have been awarded the title of curandera. Jewel Babb is particularly well-known, in part because of the publicity generated by Pat Ellis Taylor's book, *Border Healing Woman*.

Jewel Babb's story is not unlike that of many other folk healers: it wasn't until relatively late in her life that Jewel Babb discovered she had the ability to heal. Once she did, she set about doing it full time. She lives in what we would call poverty, charging nothing for her services. For the most part, she uses a combination of baths and massage. She sometimes talks about "healing with the mind," which Taylor says Mrs. Babb "visualizes as radiating from the palms of her hands when she raises them in the air, pointed in the direction of the patient."

There are many—even Mexicans and Mexican-Americans— who refer to Jewel Babb as a curandera. She, Taylor says, "satisfies the more specific expectations of her Mexican clientele, while at the same time providing a model for folk healing to which the Anglo counterculture can relate." In fact, Taylor sees Jewel Babb as "a true representative of a border culture which has provided a climate for bringing traditions together." Perhaps this is so because Jewel Babb practices, as Taylor so aptly summarizes, "a healing method which will treat the whole person."

A New Mexican friend of mine who is a modern practitioner of this ancient art is Elena Avila. She is a psychiatric nurse practitioner, writer, actor, and playwright, but most of all, she is a curandera who has been practicing for more than twenty years. Elena has garnered an international reputation as a highly competent curandera who has treated thousands for conditions of all kinds, including spiritual

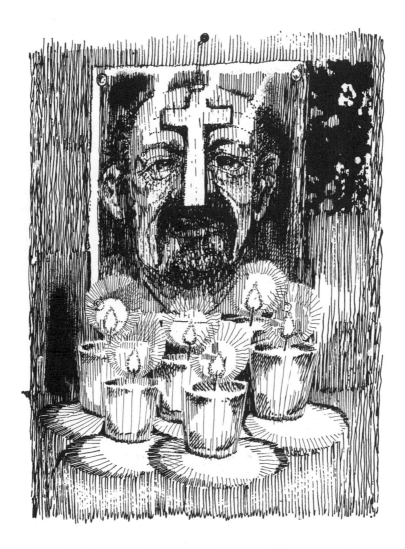

Figure 11: Modern curanderos practice many of the same techniques used by Don Pedrito, El Niño, and Teresita. They are prepared to treat their patients' physical, psychological, and spiritual needs.

illnesses such as susto and mal de ojo, as well as empacho, bilis, and muína, to name just a few. She uses an egg in her spiritual cleansing, as well as the herb *romero*. Elena has a group of followers who are apprenticing under her to learn the arts of curanderismo. I hold Elena in the greatest admiration for keeping many of the arts of Mexican folk healing alive. Like Jewel Babb, Elena works to treat the whole person, not simply the physical aspect of a patient.

This is the important thing to keep in mind about curanderismo. It does not isolate as modern science tends to; rather, it embraces. And, like an embrace, it shelters and it warms.

Chapter Ten

*Fusing Traditional and Modern Medicine**

*A*s we move into the new millennium it appears that people want to be more in charge of their own health. Throughout the world there is a growing concern that Western medicine may not provide all the answers. This may be the reason why more people are actively seeking alternative treatments to meet and maintain their holistic health needs.

Many recent Latino immigrants and undocumented workers in the United States are uninsured or underinsured, and as a result they are often forced to rely on the charity of municipal health care systems. Because of this, some may not seek care when they need it, while others have to go through the humiliating experience of waiting in overburdened emergency rooms to be treated as indigents.

When the immigrant poor come to this country, few can afford decent health insurance. Although we live in the richest country in

---

*Note: This chapter was adapted from an article that appeared in *Imagen* magazine's Special Health Issue 2003.

the world, even many Latinos whose families have been here for hundreds of years don't have adequate access to affordable health care. What I would like to do is borrow and adapt a model that I have seen at work in Mexico.

Because Mexico is a third world nation, people there have had to find other ways to get treatment for illness, particularly in the poorest rural areas where there is little access to modern health care. One way has been to continue to rely on the folk healers who have provided basic health care in rural villages for centuries.

The border country of the United States has also had these folk healers, or curanderos, who often worked long, hard hours with little rest and for little financial reward—in some cases, refusing to accept anything from their grateful clients except small gifts and enough food for a subsistence living. Curanderismo is a wonderful, ancient tradition that has roots in both the medicine of the Old World and in the wisdom of the indigenous peoples of the New World, particularly the Aztecs and Mayans, who had a vast store of knowledge about the healing and curative powers of herbs and their derivatives.

The trick is to bring curanderismo in line with conventional medicine—and vice versa, so that folk healers can work in tandem with and supplement modern medicine in the kinds of settings where people may not always have access to conventional health care. The idea is not to replace modern medicine and its life-saving technology. Instead, we want to make it possible for poor people to be able to go to someone who can tell them whether they have a condition that needs immediate medical treatment, or if they can get a folk remedy for their aches and pains.

I believe that the presence of the lay practitioner will save money within the system, when people who normally have to visit emergency rooms in county hospitals as indigents find that they can solve their medical issue more readily and cheaply by visiting a lay practitioner. Furthermore, many people might find that they do not need to visit an emergency room if the healer can help them.

The La Tranca Healing Institute in the city of Cuernavaca in the state of Morelos, Mexico, provides the model for this kind of system. Village healers and apprentices come and study with conventional doctors and nurses and experienced, certified curanderos to learn about both folk medicine and conventional medical techniques for diagnosing and treating simple illnesses. They also learn how to recognize serious conditions that require conventional medical care.

What if we set up such a system here for our own poor? What if we had a certification system to train healers in sound practices and send them out to work with the poorest of our poor? Not only could we provide people with on-the-spot help for their illnesses, the healers could also be at the forefront of important, preventative, community health initiatives and health education as well.

One of the great benefits of having Spanish-speaking lay practitioners go out into the community and offer their services is that people can more readily relate to and communicate with someone who shares their language and culture. This is a big part of why folk healers in the border region remain popular, in spite of the presence of modern medical facilities. Sometimes it gives sick people hope just to be able to talk to someone they feel understands them. In addition, the patient may more readily communicate something to a Latino healer that he would not or could not tell a doctor or nurse who didn't share his culture—in some cases, perhaps, this could save lives.

I co-teach a three-credit-hour course on the history and practices of curanderismo at the University of New Mexico's main campus in Albuquerque. Also, for the past several years, University of New Mexico students have attended classes at La Tranca Healing Institute, learning about folk healing within the context of the health care model that I hope to import to the United States. I envision folding these courses into future pilot efforts toward building a new health care model in the U.S. My hope is that training lay practitioners alongside doctors and nurses will become part of standard medical school curricula nationwide. To help as many people as we can, we have to dream big.

Chapter Eleven

Further Reading Pertaining to Curanderismo

There isn't a great deal of material available about curanderismo, and some of it may be difficult to find. I have made a list of some of the books that have appealed to me as well as those I have quoted at various places in this text. Most are nonfiction, but there are a few novels that have scenes or plots involving curanderismo and ought to be mentioned. One such is **Caldo Largo** by Earle Thompson (Signet New American Library, 1976). This well-written, hard-hitting adventure story is set in the ports of South Texas and Mexico. It is still in print in paperback, available from Carroll & Graf Publishers. Another, though lesser known, novel is **Bless Me, Ultima** by Rudolfo A. Anaya (Warner Books, 1994), winner of the Second Annual *Premio Quinto Sol* National Chicano literary award. It is available in paper from Amazon, Barnes and Noble, and other major booksellers.

Others, in no particular order, are:

Cooking and Curing With Mexican Herbs by Dolores L. Latorre (Encino Press, 1977). This text, based on research done in Mexico, mentions quite a few folk ills that are ignored elsewhere. It is also an excellent and handsomely put together cookbook.

Woman Who Glows in the Dark: Curandera Reveals Traditional Aztec Secrets of Physical and Spiritual Health by Elena Avila (with Joy Parker) (Jeremy Tarcher/Putnam reprint edition, 2000). Elena is a friend of mine who does powerful one-woman performances about the art of curanderismo and about her own life and how she became a healer. Her book is well worth taking the time to read, and if you ever get a chance to see her perform, seize it.

Curanderismo: Mexican-American Folk Psychiatry by Ari Kiev (The Free Press, 1968). Kiev examines curanderismo from the point of view of a psychiatrist. In fact, he relates many of the folk illnesses to psychiatric disorders. He is very good at analyzing the way curanderismo works and why.

Curanderismo by Robert T. Trotter and Juan Antonio Chavira (University of Georgia Press, 1981). This book was done as part of a grant given to acquaint health care professionals in regions with a high Mexican-American population with practices of curanderismo. It shows the way the traditional folk methods complement their formal counterparts. Its descriptions of the rituals are particularly good.

Folk Practices in Northern Mexico, Isabel Truesdell Kelly (University of Texas Press, 1965). This is a hard book to find, but it focuses on beliefs relating to health. Although the study was done in Mexico, the findings also apply to Mexican-Americans.

Stories That Must Not Die by Juan Sauvageau (Oasis Press, 1957–6). These four volumes recount stories and legends collected by Sauvageau and his students from the South Texas and Rio Grande Valley areas. They are presented in both English and Spanish, side by side, and each tale is followed by questions to aid discussion. In this way, they are effective classroom books as well as just plain interesting reading.

Discovering Folklore Through Community Resources, edited by Magdalena Benavides Sumpter was published in 1978 by the Development and Assessment Center for Bilingual Education in Austin, Texas. It is an elementary school text put together "in order to rediscover and preserve a part of the culture of the Mexican-American as it relates to folkloric tradition." It is extremely simplified, of course, and valuable particularly to the parent who wishes to introduce his children to curanderismo and its practices.

The Healer of Los Olmos and Other Mexican Lore, edited by Wilson M. Hudson (Southern Methodist University Press, 1975). This is one of the marvelous books published by the Texas Folklore Society. The section that deals with Don Pedrito Jaramillo is the most famous and it was compiled by Ruth Dodson, who "decided to collect and write down the stories the people told about this man." It is a valuable resource and even contains photographs of Don Pedrito.

Don Pedrito Jaramillo: Curandero, a bilingual series of descriptions and anecdotes about the healer of Los Olmos, was written and published by an amateur folklorist, Ruth Dodson, in the 1930s and republished by her niece, Henrietta Newbury, in 1994. Some of the stories it contains are quite fascinating. Dodson reputedly became interested in the great healer when she met a child who had been cured of her clubfeet by Don Pedrito.

Niño Fidencio: A Heart Thrown Open, by Dore Gardner and Kay F. Turner (Museum of New Mexico Press, 1992). This collection of interviews and photographs by Gardner with an essay by Turner provides a visual and textual documentation of the powerful phenomenon of the great festivals of the fidencistas in Espinazo, Nuevo Leon, Mexico. I have attended these festivals myself, and I found them to be, quite literally, life-changing events for me.

Teresita by William Curry Holden (Stemmer House, 1978). In novelistic fashion, Holden pieces together and makes intensely

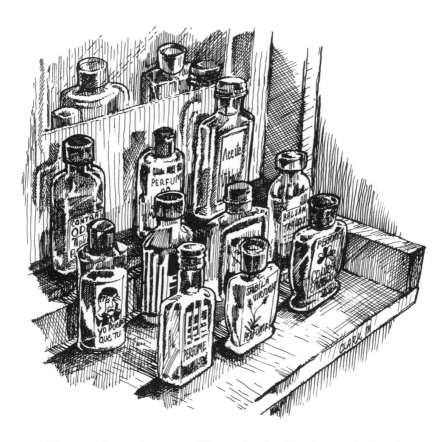

Figure 12: Curanderos use different levels of healing including the spiritual, mental, and material levels. For the material level, they can use magical perfumes, liniments, and herbal tinctures and oils.

dramatic the story of Teresa Urrea, the Mexican curandera and psychic. Holden researched this subject for more than twenty years.

Border Healing Woman by Pat Ellis Taylor (University of Texas Press, 1981). A very feeling collection of interviews with Jewel Babb, an Anglo healer whom some say has earned the title of curandera. Taylor, whose appreciation of Jewel Babb shines through on every page, is the perfect counterpoint to her subject.

Arigo: Surgeon of the Rusty Knife by John G. Fuller (Crowell, 1974). I mention this book only because it is such a fascinating case, relaying as it does the story of a simple Brazilian peasant who, in a trance state, took on the spirit—and the abilities—of a German doctor and who performed incredible feats of healing. The word curandero when used in Brazil, interestingly, is a pejorative term, always, the author says, connoting witchcraft.

Sastun: My Apprenticeship with a Maya Healer by Rosita Arvigo (Harper, 1994). This book chronicles the relationship between one of the last great practitioners of the ancient art of Mayan medicine and an American who moved from Chicago to Belize to open a medical clinic in the jungle. A fascinating account of the meeting of two cultures and people from vastly different backgrounds, and a tribute to the ancient medicinal arts of the indigenous peoples of Latin America.

Part Two

*Green Medicine:
Traditional
Mexican-American
Herbs and Remedies*

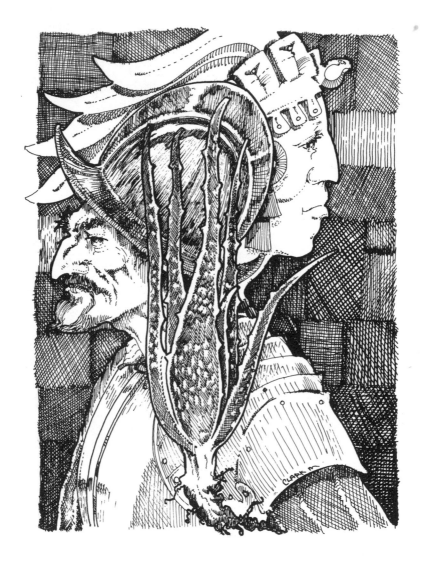

Figure 13: The Aloe Vera, *Zabila*, is an example of a plant introduced by the Spaniards to the indigenous people of the New World.

Introduction

There is a lot of interest in green medicine. I know, because I have been asked to take my "Traveling Medicine Show," a lecture on Mexican-American herbal remedies, not just all over the Southwest, but to other regions as well. And I have been asked to appear on various television shows and have been interviewed by newspaper reporters more often than I can easily remember. That is the sort of interest that the subject of herbal medicine inspires.

There is a lot of interest in reading about the subject, too. In fact, I have never appeared before a group without someone in the audience asking me if I have a book about herbal medicine that they could buy. That is why I decided to write this one: to serve as an introduction to the subject of green medicine, much as my "Traveling Medicine Show" does.

Oh, there are books about the subject, to be sure. Most of these, however, are written by scholars for scholars. They don't take into account the average person who just wants to get acquainted with what can be a very complicated subject. And those books that are more general are just that: too general. They include remedies from all over, not just those used by Mexican-Americans.

This is, of course, the portion of the subject that interests me. I am a Mexican-American who has always lived in the Southwest, where curanderismo, or folk healing, flourishes. I grew up with many of these remedies, and even though I went on to earn a doctorate and become a vice president at a university, I have not abandoned many of them, particularly the teas.

But even those that I, personally, do not use haven't ceased to fascinate me. It is my pleasure to share them all with you now—the green medicine that is part of curanderismo.

Chapter Twelve

Green Medicine: An Introduction

$\mathbf{I}$f I were to use the word "medicine," and ask you to picture something illustrating that word in your mind, what would you think of? Chances are you would think of a patent medicine you might find on the supermarket shelf: Alka Seltzer or Pepto Bismol or maybe a cold remedy like NyQuil. Then again, you might envision one of the little plastic bottles that pharmacists use for prescription drugs, the kind with the impossible-to-open childproof lids and the brightly colored capsules inside. Or maybe you would think of the vaccination that you got before you took that trip abroad a few years back. In any case, if I were to use the word, "medicine," it probably wouldn't conjure up the image of a plant.

Many modern medicines, however, come from plants. Most people know that digitalis comes from the Foxglove plant, which was used for heart ailments long before anyone had figured out why it worked. A lot of people know, too, that the chemical that is found in curare is a potent anesthetic. But let me give you another example that in many ways serves to illustrate one major premise of this book.

In the early 1600s, when the Peruvian Indians seemed to be the only people who were not dying of malaria, it was discovered that they were treating the illness with a tea made from the ground bark of the *Chinchona* tree. This "Peruvian bark," as it later was called in Europe, contains the substance known as quinine.

Eventually, as often happens with remedies derived from plants, synthetic versions of quinine were developed and these superceded the botanical remedy. This is why the word "medicine" so infrequently makes us think of plants. But interestingly, in this case, the original remedy staged an unexpected comeback when a strain of malaria surfaced during the Vietnam war. This strain proved resistant to the synthetics that had been developed in the lab.

Was there anything that would cure this new strain? Yes, the original botanical remedy: Peruvian bark—from the Chinchona tree.

What does this demonstrate? That the old remedies derived from plants do have a solid medical basis. And that they are sometimes better than the synthetics derived from them.

But the story of Peruvian bark is illustrative in still another way. For instance, though malaria was the world's number one killer disease when a Jesuit first publicized the Peruvian Indian cure, the medical profession in Europe went out of its way to disprove the claims that were made for it.

A few physicians, for example, tested the bark with disastrous results. It was too dangerous to use, they concluded. Plus the remedy didn't have the sanction of appearing in a text by Galen—a famous physician of ancient Rome—who had codified his cures by writing them down in what was to become the bible of the medical profession. Pretty soon someone came on the scene with a secret mixture that was supposed to be better than the remedy that the Indians used. Everyone ignored Peruvian bark and chose this (probably much more expensive) medicine instead. After the death of the person who concocted it, its ingredients were revealed. And, of course, the main one was Peruvian bark.

We can learn a lot from this, not atypical, example.

But herbal cures today are being given more credence than they were, say, thirty years ago. I doubt that we will return to the era when physicians routinely took courses in botany in order to study the *Materia Medica*, but, largely because of the mounting popularity of the holistic movement—e.g., the theory of looking at a person's illness in the context of his beliefs, his lifestyle, his diet, and so on—herbal cures are once again on the rise.

In the Mexican-American tradition, herbal cures—or green medicine, as it is sometimes called—have always been prominent. In large measure, these are used to treat minor ailments and are no more than inexpensive and readily accessible home remedies or, as they are called in Spanish, *remedios caseros*. But more importantly, herbal cures are part of an elaborate system of folk healing which Mexican-Americans call curanderismo.

You have only to look at the word to know—or at least to come up with a very good guess at—what it means. It derives from the Spanish verb curar, to cure. And a practitioner of curanderismo— a healer—would be a curandero or a curandera (the former, if a man; the latter, if a woman). Interestingly, female healers are as prevalent as male.

But curanderos, like physicians, have specialties. There are materias or espiritistas—those who are mediums between this world and the beyond; there are parteras, or midwives; and señoras, who foretell the future by reading cards. Finally, and of greatest interest to us here, there are the *yerberas*, or herbalists. They are the ones who are most likely to employ green medicine to its fullest. Many of the vendors who bring herbs to the marketplaces in Mexico are, in fact, curanderos and yerberas.

Is curanderismo dying out? It does not seem to be. In many American cities far from Mexico—even Detroit and Chicago—there are enormous numbers of Mexican-Americans whose presence keeps it alive. In Chicago, for instance, there is even a shrine to the famous Mexican curandero, Niño Fidencio, and each year, people from Chicago and from other cities all over the United States journey to Espinazo, Mexico, where El Niño lived and healed. One might say that, far from dying out, curanderismo thrives.

And those in formal medicine have begun to respect it, too. In one Denver mental health facility, for example, there is a curandera on the staff. But more and more, too, formal medicine—because of the aforementioned holistic or naturopathic swing—has begun to resemble curanderismo. For example, a 1983 article in a national women's magazine touted something called therapeutic touching as a medical breakthrough. A form of this has been practiced by curanderos for centuries! Another popular magazine, just a month later, had a page devoted to the medicinal value of oil extracted from evening primrose. As *flor de San Juan*, evening primrose had long been part of curanderismo!

Some social scientists say that naturopathy is not merely a fad but a reasonable reaction against the technological brand of medicine we see everywhere around us: laser surgery, organ transplants, battery-powered limbs, and even electronic mood equalizers. All of this is on the one hand, marvelous, and on the other, off-putting in the extreme. Most people, after gasping in awe, cannot help but say, "Wait a minute, what about us? As people?" Thus begins the search for something with deeper roots.

Well, the Mexican and Mexican-American cultures have, in fact, never let go of what some cultures have only begun to realize is of importance. This insistence on the human element is probably what has kept curanderismo from fading away all these years.

It is true, of course, that some practices have changed. *Hueseros,* or bonesetters, for instance, have all but disappeared, replaced by physicians who are more effective at setting bones. But for other ailments, the formal practitioner is, well, too formal. He requires that an appointment be made. He requires a rather high payment, too. And in all likelihood, he doesn't speak Spanish. He might also be in another part of town. The typical curandero will have none of these drawbacks: he will be, most likely, a neighbor or at least a trusted

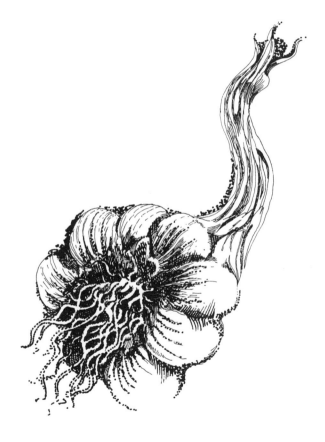

Figure 14: With its antibacterial and anti-inflammatory properties, garlic is used for burns, abrasions, earaches, and insect bites.

member of the patient's community. He will, therefore, speak Spanish. He will understand the social and psychological context in which the patient has developed the disease. And his cure—because he believes that it is dictated by God—will not be costly. In most cases, it will cost whatever the patient deems it to be worth.

The element of belief of the patient will, of course, play a part in the cure. Even the stuffiest formal medical doctor cannot deny that it always does, whether the patient is treated in a *barrio* in San Antonio, Albuquerque, Chicago, Phoenix, or Denver, or at a shock trauma center somewhere else. Expectation of a cure is always important.

But some remedies will work just as well without the element of faith. Mexican housewives, for instance, used to scrape the mold off tortillas and feed it to those suffering from infection. How were they to know that the folk medicine they were offering would later be called penicillin? There are many common substances used medicinally—garlic, for example—which, after scientific study, have been found to contain known healing agents.

But Mexicans and Mexican-Americans do not have to be convinced of this. They have for so long relied on herbal reliefs that, if anything, it seems odd not to rely on them. Evelyne Winter, who gathered a list of folk remedies from all over Mexico in the 1950s, reported, for example, that one of her informants had a hard time convincing a cab driver that she wasn't daft when she admitted to drinking tea just for the pleasure of drinking tea, rather than to effect a cure for some ailment or other!

Chapter Thirteen

A Brief History of Green Medicine

Two scholars from Pan American University studied curanderismo and concluded that it derived from or is influenced by six separate elements:

Judeo-Christian religion, symbols, and rituals
Early Arabic medicine and health practices
Medieval and later European witchcraft
Native American herbal lore
Modern Western beliefs about psychic phenomena
Modern medicine.

Of these six, some pertain to green medicine more clearly than others. An understanding of the Native American herbal lore—that is, those remedies that the Indians of Mexico were practicing at the time of the Spanish conquest—and a brief examination of the reference to early Arabic medicine is sufficient to provide a simplified view of herbal healing, not just as it is practiced by the curanderos, but as it is handed down in Mexican-American families from one generation to the next.

Let us consider first the Aztec culture, which, more than any other Indian culture in Mexico, including the Mayan, Toltec, and Zapotec-Mixtec, influenced the herbal aspects of curanderismo.

At the time of the Spanish conquest, the Aztec civilization was remarkably advanced. There was socialized medicine, for example, including hospitals in various cities throughout the Aztec empire where injured warriors could be treated free of cost. There was great emphasis on sanitation, not merely from the personal standpoint, but also regarding public sanitation as it affected public health. And there was ongoing botanical research for medical purposes.

The Huaxtepec garden, for example, devoted entirely to this purpose, had a seven mile circumference! Montezuma's gardens are described by Cervantes de Salazar in his 1554 book titled *Dialogues*, and here we learn that there were some two thousand species of trees, shrubs, and herbs for healing.

Unfortunately, the Spanish friars destroyed all of the Aztec's own written records of botanical successes and failures. The Aztecs, after all, were considered savages by these priests. What we do know of Aztec civilization was documented by men commissioned by more enlightened members of the government of Spain especially so that Aztec medical contributions would not be entirely lost!

It is no wonder, though, that few realize how advanced the Aztecs were. But even some who should know better tacitly insult the mighty Aztec nation. Consider the opinion inherent in this passage, for instance, from the pen of George Foster, a scholar writing in the *Journal of American Folklore*. The Aztec understanding of medicine, he writes, "was probably not greatly inferior to that of Spanish physicians." This offhand dismissal of Aztec achievement fails to take into account all of the things I mentioned earlier: the hospitals, the public sanitation, and even documented surgical successes!

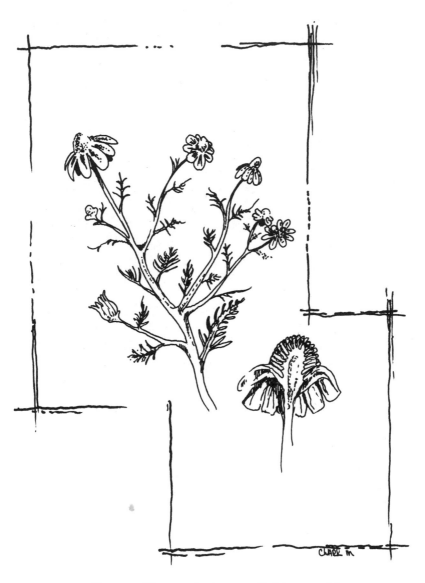

Figure 15: Chamomile (manzanilla) is a soothing
sedative and also aids digestion.

This is not to say that the men who came to Mexico from Spain brought nothing. Some items they are known to have introduced include chamomile, onions, garlic, rosemary, lemons, and oranges, to name a few. Most importantly, however, they brought with them a medical theory that pervades curanderismo even today.

This is the theory of "the humors," first introduced by Hippocrates, the Greek physician who is called the "father of medicine."

The theory of the humors presumes that there are four liquids in the human body: blood, phlegm, yellow bile, and black bile. These are allied with the elements:

Blood, allied to air, is hot and moist
Phlegm, allied to water, is cold and moist
Yellow bile, allied to fire, is hot and dry
Black bile, allied to earth, is cold and dry.

Physical ailments, and even the various dispositions that people have, were said to be caused by the imbalance or disproportion of the humors. Medicine, then, was an attempt to restore the balance. This theory of the humors, though, is not peculiar to curanderismo. It plays a large part in all traditional healing systems. While it originated with the Greeks and Romans, it was transmitted via the Arabs and thus reached Spain. In those days, it was part of formal—as opposed to folk—medicine, with all medical practice being a matter of restoring the body's fundamental harmony.

Formal medicine was very early entrenched in Mexico, by the way. A chair of medicine was established at the University of Mexico in 1580, and before then, curing was taught on a more casual basis at the Colegio de Santa Cruz in Tlaltelolco.

Chapter Fourteen

Where to Get the Herbs

O riginally, herbal medicine was the only possible choice. There were no drugstores. If aloe vera was plentiful in a given area, it was chosen over *maguey*, and vice versa. Availability is one reason there are so many alternatives listed for a given ailment—occasionally an illness struck and one had to cast about for an herb to cure it.

Eventually, botanical gardens—not necessarily on the scale of the Aztec gardens, but planned herbal plots nonetheless—were standard. Even today, some easy-to-grow herbs are cultivated, even in city apartments. Aloe vera, for instance, flourishes as a house-plant, and mint, parsley, and similar herbs can be grown in the backyard or even in a window box.

And, of course, herbs still grow in the wild.

The most common method of getting the herbs used in green medicine, however, is to buy them. Because many are used in cook-ing, they will often be found on the spice shelf of any supermarket. Other more esoteric herbs can be found in health food stores, usu-ally as bottled tinctures with an alcohol base. Only occasionally—

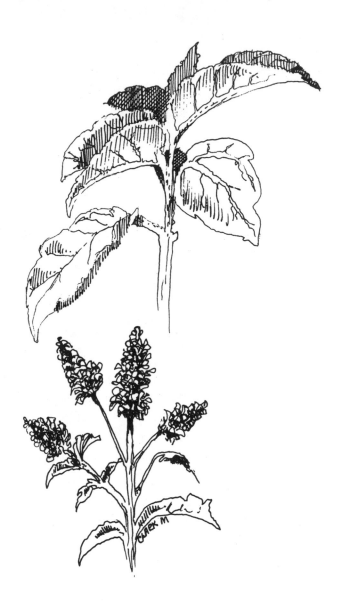

Figure 16: Mint (yerba buena) relieves stomachaches and nausea, and it also restores energy.

say in the case of powdered garlic—will the method of preparing herbs for sale alter their healing potential.

Those who live in cities near the Mexican border or in cities with a large Mexican-American population will usually find these herbs on sale in their neighborhoods. In most cases, they will be bundled, wrapped in plastic, and tagged with the names in Spanish, just as they are given in italics in the glossary of this book. In these stores that sell herbs—*yerberías*, *hierberías*, or *botánicas*—it is frequently possible to get advice about the use or preparation of a given herb, though the proprietors must take care not to violate the law by "practicing medicine without a license." Usually you will be told that "one often uses . . ." or "it is sometimes recommended that you . . ." much as I have done in this book.

In Mexico itself, most marketplaces or *mercados* will have a yerbería with bulk or prepacked herbs. In many areas, too, there is often an open air market with makeshift stalls where herbs gathered from the plains and mountains will be sold. And remember, often the vendors are curanderos who can give advice on the use of the herbs they sell. These yerberías are becoming popular at weekend flea markets throughout the Southwest in communities with large Mexican-American populations.

Chapter Fifteen

Preparing Herbs for Use

Herbal remedies are most often taken as teas, in which case they are decocted or infused—terms to be explained later. Chamomile is probably the best known example of an herb used as a tea.

Occasionally, however, herbs are burned and either smoked or used as an incense. In the latter category, juniper is often used. Many of the herbs that are smoked are illegal (marijuana) or dangerous (jimson weed), but some are not: eucalyptus or mullein are two good examples.

Sometimes, too, the herbs are prepared in tincture, microdoses, or maceration. All three of these methods seem to concentrate the qualities of the herb so prepared.

Herbs can be made into a poultice or plaster to be applied directly to the skin. The mustard plaster is probably the one most people are familiar with.

But washes, too, are popular, either applied to the skin or used to rinse the mouth. A rosemary wash, prepared exactly as tea to be consumed, is probably the best example.

Usually when an herb comes with instructions that it be brewed as a tea, the method of preparation will be infusion or decoction. An infusion requires that boiling water be poured over the herb and that it steeps for at least five minutes in a covered container. A decoction requires that the herb be placed into water that is boiling and then be permitted to simmer (not boil) for at least five minutes. In either case, the herb is strained away and the resulting liquid is the tea, however it is used.

A maceration is made by placing the herb in water and leaving it for at least ten hours, but often as long as a week. The constituents will separate and the thin top layer can be poured off. The resulting mixture, after the herb has been strained away, is taken in the appropriate dosage.

A tincture is prepared by mashing the herb and then soaking it in ninety-six proof Mexican alcohol, vodka, or wine in a darkened place such as a closet. Usually a week is sufficient. Before the tincture is used, it is strained.

A microdose is a tincture diluted with water that acts as a homeopathic medication and is often used by those not tolerant to alcohol.

One general rule that should be followed no matter what mode of preparation is chosen is this: never use aluminum or Teflon when preparing herbs. Glass is best, though steel is acceptable.

It is also wise to remember that dried herbs are stronger—sometimes even twice as strong—as freshly picked herbs.

It is very difficult to give exact dosages when dealing with herbs. The potency of the plant can change with the size of the plant, the soil in which it has grown, and a host of other variable elements. This, in fact, is one reason plant remedies were eventually synthesized in the lab: they could thus be made predictable. In general, however, a tablespoon of dried herb to a cup of liquid is a good starting point whatever the method of preparation. Herbs are potent. Just keep in mind the tiny amount of tea in an average teabag!

Chapter Sixteen

A Few Cautions

Any book about herbs is bound to be filled with cautions. Herbs are, after all, potent medicine. It is possible to overdose on herbs just as it is to overdose on street drugs. In addition, many plants have poisonous parts. It may be perfectly safe to eat the leaves of a plant, for example, and deadly to eat the blossoms, or vice versa. Or the plant may be perfectly safe if eaten fresh, but become poisonous as it wilts.

It is no wonder, then, that books about herbs have to contain a lot of warnings. In fact, to be on the safe side, consider this statement an inflexible rule: *never* eat, chew, or drink tea brewed from any part of an unknown plant.

For example, some plants with poisonous berries are mistletoe, holly, and any variety of ivy. Plants with poisonous leaves include azalea, lily of the valley, and elephant ears. Plants with poisonous roots or bulbs include iris, daffodil, and violet. Some plants have poisonous stems, vines, or seeds. In this category are potato, tomato, cherry, rhubarb, and hydrangea. Still others—peach and apricot, to name two—have poisonous pits.

Herbal medicine, obviously, can be far from benign!

The Brooklyn Botanic Garden in New York illustrated this very well one year by exhibiting a surprising array of plants that can cause harm. These ranged from English ivy to yew. (The leaves and seeds of yew, if eaten, can cause heart failure!)

And from an historic standpoint, the toxic characteristics of some plants have provoked some really interesting speculation. For example, there is one theory that the Salem witches weren't witches after all, but had eaten an hallucinogenic substance similar to LSD. They are thought to have consumed St. Anthony's fire, a fungus that grows on grain—especially rye.

Also, every now and then, dangerous ingredients are included in pre-packaged herbal remedies. For example, one supplier of "folk" medicine produced two cures for empacho called "Greta" and "Azarcón." Greta proved to have a base of lead monoxide and Azarcón was 90 percent lead tetroxide. Both were extremely toxic and were in regular use in a number of Mexican and Mexican-American homes! Though they were originally blended to cure empacho, which is similar to intestinal blockage, they were being used to treat headache and even menstrual disorders.

Lead monoxide—and Greta, when analyzed, proved to have 90 to 98 percent of this substance as its base—changes to lead chloride at stomach temperatures and, because of this, is readily absorbed into the bloodstream. The base metal of Azarcón did not convert to lead chloride and was less dangerous. But both, if ingested over long periods of time, would cause lead poisoning.

Lead poisoning can kill but more often those who survive are left severely retarded or handicapped in other ways.

It is thought that Greta and Azarcón became popular because they are similar in color to a remedy used by curanderos: saffron or, in Spanish, *azafrán*. The pre-packaged formulas seem to be attempts to copy the folk remedy for empacho, but alas, in this case, with disastrous or even lethal results.

Still another caution is not to rely on folk remedies and neglect standard medical treatment. Indeed, folk and formal medicine should complement each other. It is not unusual, nowadays, for a curandero to refer a patient to a licensed medical practitioner.

Chapter Seventeen

Important Terms

There are a lot of terms used to describe what a given substance does that are unfamiliar to the general reading public. I have defined them—at least on the first use—in my glossary. If you are planning to read other herbals (what glossaries describing herbs and their effects are often called), you will encounter them regularly and ought to memorize them.

Analgesic: Something that takes pain away, but does not cause loss of consciousness. An analgesic may be swallowed or rubbed on the skin or be used as a gargle. The effect categorizes it. Willow bark (*raíz de sáuce*) falls into this category.

Anaphrodisiac: Something that lessens sexual desire. Its opposite, of course, is an aphrodisiac. Lettuce (*lechuga*), for instance, and camphor (*alcanfor*), are thought to be anaphrodisiacs.

Anesthetic: This can refer to a substance that causes loss of consciousness, but then again, it could also refer to one that doesn't. Oil of cloves (*aceite de clavo*) would be an example of the latter. An anesthetic kills sensation.

Anodyne: Can refer to a painkiller or merely to something that soothes. Aloe vera (zabila), for example, can be an anodyne for someone with sunburn, as can papaya for someone who had been stung by a jellyfish.

Anthelmintic: This means that it eliminates worms. Pumpkin seeds (*pepitas*) are the most renowned anthelmintic.

Antidote: This is a substance that counteracts the effects of a poison. Musk mallow (*malva*) is used as an antidote for snake bites.

Antiemetic: Something that stops vomiting and nausea. Mint (yerba buena), for instance, is antiemetic.

Antihydrotic: This is the opposite of a diaphoretic. It refers to a substance that dries up bodily fluids. Sage (*salvia*) is used to dry up secretions.

Antipyretic: Something that reduces fever. Elder flowers (*flor de saúco*) are used for those with fever.

Antiseptic: Something that stops the growth of microorganisms (germs) and therefore is likely to prevent infection. Garlic (*ajo*) and oshá (*chuchupate*) are used as antiseptics.

Antispasmodic: Stops muscle spasms and cramps. Valerian (*valeriana*), for instance, is a known antispasmodic.

Aphrodisiac: Something that increases sexual desire. *Damiana* is used as an aphrodisiac.

Astringent: Something that is applied to contract pores. Sage (salvia), and oak (*encino*) are used as a skin astringent.

Carminative: Also called an antiflatulent, this is something that gets rid of gas. Fennel seeds (*hinojo*) and aniseeds (anís) are said to be carminatives.

Cathartic: Causes bowels to evacuate. Another word for a laxative or purgative. Bearberry (*cascara sagrada*) is used as a gentle laxative.

Coagulant: Causes clotting. The Mexican dayflower (*yerba del pollo*) is used to stop bleeding.

Demulcent: A substance that soothes an inflamed area. Aloe vera, for example, is a demulcent.

Diaphoretic: Something that increases sweating. Borage (*boraja*) and Mexican tea (*epazote*) induce sweating.

Disinfectant: An antiseptic or a substance used to kill germs. Creosote bush (*gobernadora*) is used to disinfect wounds.

Diuretic: Something that increases the flow of urine. Cornsilk (*barbas de elote*) is used as a diuretic.

Emetic: A substance taken to induce vomiting. In large quantities, nutmeg (*nuez moscada*) can induce vomiting, as can violet (*violeta*) root.

Emmenagogue: A substance that stimulates menstrual flow. Mexican tea (epazote) is used for delayed menstruation.

Emollient: Something applied externally to soften and soothe. Aloe vera (zabila) is applied to the skin to soothe skin problems.

Expectorant: A substance taken to expel mucous from the respiratory tract. Mountain balm (*yerba santa*) and mullein (*gordolobo*) are expectorants.

Germicide: An antiseptic or disinfectant—that is, something to kill germs. Thyme (*tomillo*) is used as an antibacterial agent.

Liniment: A medicinal fluid applied to the skin as an anodyne.

Purgative: Something that causes the bowels to evacuate. Another term for a laxative or cathartic. Bearberry (cascara sagrada) is a mild laxative.

Restorative: Something taken to renew energy. Mint tea is thought to be a restorative.

Sedative: Something that calms and reduces nervousness. Passion flower (*passiflora*) is used for nervousness.

Soporific: The opposite of a stimulant, a soporific induces sleep. Tea made from orange blossoms (*azahár*), for example, is said to be a soporific, as is chamomile (manzanilla).

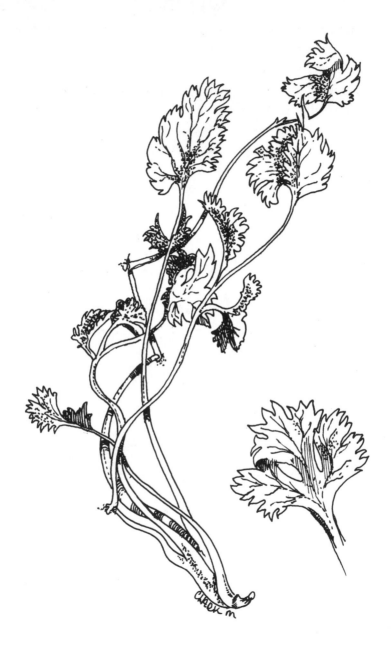

Figure 17: Parsley (*perejil*) relieves menstrual cramps and insect bites.

Stimulant: A restorative. Damian (damiana) is a stimulant.

Styptic: An astringent applied to stop bleeding. Lemon (*limón*), for instance, is a styptic.

Tranquilizer: Something that calms. A sedative. Valerian (valeriana) has a sedative effect.

Unguent: A soothing or healing salve. Many herbs are used in salves.

Vulnerary: A substance that promotes healing. *Tepezcohuite* promotes healing and works to regenerate skin.

Chapter Eighteen

Keeping Green
Medicine Alive

I hope that the information presented in this section has given you a greater appreciation of green medicine, which has been around since the beginning of time and has evolved through the centuries.

The valuable knowledge of herbs has basically been passed from mother to daughter and from father to son. Nowadays, however, many second and third generation Mexican-Americans are forgetting the traditional use of green medicine. For this reason, I have chosen to elaborate on the subject here.

The Mexican and Mexican-American practice of green medicine has been of special interest to me and I hope to help, in some small way, in keeping that knowledge alive.

It has always been a source of pride to me—as it should to everyone with Mexican ancestry—that Mexican-American herbal medicine is the product of such a rich blend of European, Asian, and native Indian knowledge and tradition.

Perhaps it is this that has sparked the interest in both the historical and therapeutic aspects of herbal medicine now being shown by those who are not members of the Mexican-American community.

I hope that this book will answer the need for information on this subject. Much of it is not readily available, and often, when it can be found, is addressed to the scholar or botanist rather than the average person with an interest in herbal medicine.

This book then, like the herbs and folk healers that are its subject, is also a remedy of sorts.

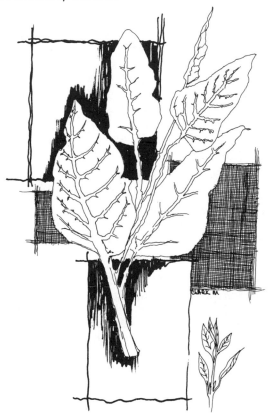

Figure 18: Sage (*salvia*) is an effective mouthwash for sore gums.

Chapter Nineteen

Further Reading Pertaining to Green Medicine

Should you wish to continue reading about folk medicine or herbal healing the following is a list of books that might interest you. This list is not meant to be exhaustive.

Las Yerbas de la Gente: A Study of Hispano-American Medicinal Plants, Karen Cowan Ford (University of Michigan, 1975). This is an extensive listing of various herbs used medicinally by Mexican Americans and other Hispanics. I found it invaluable in crosschecking my herbal references. It also emphasizes in some cases the sheer variety of different species that are listed under the same common Spanish name.

Medicinal Plants of the Mountain West, Michael Moore (Museum of New Mexico Press, 1979, revised 2003). This book usually lists plants by their common English names first. Michael Moore is in many ways the dean of all medicinal herbalists of the West and the Southwest. Given the wide variety of plants falling under a given common name I sometimes used his books to help me determine exactly which species listed under a given broadly used common name would be most likely to appear in the Southwestern region, from which much of this herbal wisdom emanates.

Los Remedios: Traditional Herbal Remedies of the Southwest, Michael Moore (Red Crane Books, 1990). See above entry. This book lists the Spanish names as primary, and covers a somewhat different range of herbs. But it was just as invaluable to me as the book listed above.

Green Pharmacy, Barbara Griggs (Viking, 1981). This is a history of herbal medicine, including the disputes and controversies that have surrounded it through the ages. It makes no mention of curanderismo, but does include an account of the way in which the birth control pill was derived from the Mexican yam.

Herbs and Things, Jeanne Rose (Workman, 1972). A charming and informal herbal which includes such things as herbal baths, veterinary potions, sachets and potpourris, and a section titled "Various Forbidden Secrets," e.g., about some witchcraft ceremonies.

Infusions of Healing: A Treasury of Mexican-American Herbal Remedies, Jolie Davidow (Simon & Schuster, 1999). This is an excellent herbal, listing many herbs with Spanish, English, and botanical names, plus parts of the plant used, plant properties, and treatments.

Mexico's Ancient and Native Remedies, Evelyne Winter (Editorial Fournier, 1968). This sounds more promising than it is. It is not a collection of old remedies, but rather, a collection of the remedies of various people Winter encounters.

Grandmother's Tea, Joe Graham (Institute of Texan Cultures, 1979). This was really designed for school children and provides a very elementary approach to herbal healing in the Mexican-American culture. There is a slide show that goes with the text, however, and a good bibliography.

Folk Medicine and Herbal Healing, G. Meyer, Kenneth Blum, and John G. Cull, eds. (Charles C. Thomas, 1981). It will not be easy to find this book, even in libraries. It is a collection of articles on the subject in "an effort to present . . . the current status of folk healing and herbal medicine." The editors are based in San Antonio, and, though their intention is to discuss all folk systems rather than just curanderismo, many of the articles have a Mexican-American slant.

Cooking and Curing with Mexican Herbs, Dolores L. Latorre (Encino Press, 1977). This beautiful book is illustrated with wood-cuts. About two-thirds of it could be called a cookbook. The healing portion lists conditions and diseases and then the herbs that are said to cure them.

The De la Cruz-Badiano Aztec herbal of 1552, Martin de la Cruz (Dover 2000). This edition of the famous Aztec herbal of 1552, the

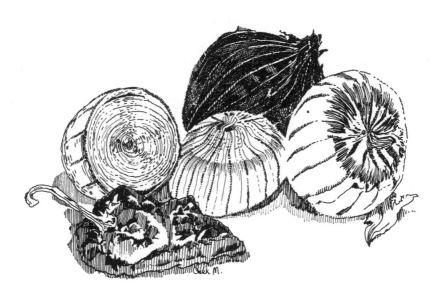

Figure 19: Onion (*cebolla*) is said to effect a number of different cures including bronchial complaints, while cayenne pepper (*cucurbita*) purportedly stops bleeding.

Codex Badiano, was originally put out in the 1930s; Dover, known for reprint editions of classic works, has reissued it. This book is one of the great works in the annals of early ethnobotanical research, essentially preserving for later generations a remnant of the vast medicinal herbal knowledge of the Aztec empire of Mexico.

Appendix: Spanish Language Listing of Plant Names

Note: Common Spanish language names of the plants named in the glossary of herbs in this book are given here first in boldface roman type, followed by their common English names in non-boldface roman type, and finally by their botanical names in italics.

Acedera, Sorrell, *Rumex acetosa*

Aconito, Monkshood (Wolfsbane), *Aconitum sp.*

Agave (Maguey), Century Plant, Mescal, *Agave sp.*

Agenjo (Ajenjo), Wormwood, *Artemisia mexicana*

Ajenjibre (Jengibre), Ginger, *Zingiber offinale*

Ajenjo (Agenjo), Wormwood, *Artemisia mexicana*

Ajo, Garlic, *Allium sativum*

Albahaca, Basil (Sweet Basil), *Ocimum basilicum*

Alcanfor, Camphor, *Cinnamomum camphora*

Alhucema (Espliego, Lavanda), Lavender, *Lavandula sp.*

Altimisa (Zizim, Zitzim), Mugwort (Mountain Mugwort), *Artemisia franserioides*

Altimisa Mexicana (Santa Maria), Feverfew, *Chrysanthemum parthenium*

Añil (Jiguilete), Indigo, *Indigofera anil, Indigofera sp.*

Anís, Aniseed, *Pimpinella anisum*

Anís Estrella, Star Anise, *Illicum verum*

Arbol de la Cera, Bayberry, *Myrica californica, M. cerifera*

Aristoloquia (Moja de Guaco), Birthwort, *Aristolochia clematitis,*
    A. serpentaria, A. tomentosa, Aristolochia sp.

Arnica, Arnica, *Arnica cardifolia*

Arnica Mexicana, Camphor Weed, *Heterotheca sp.*

Barbas de Elote (Pelos de Elote), Cornsilk, *Zea mays*

Berro, Watercress, *Nasturtium officinale*

Borraja, Borage, *Borago officinalis*

Buganbilia (Buganvilla), Bougainvilla, *Bougainvillea spectabilis*

Cachana, Gay Feather, Blazing Star, *Liatris punctada*

Calabaza, Pumpkin, *Cucurbita pepo*

Caléndula, Marigold, *Calendula officinalis*

Canaigre, Red Dock, *Rumex hymenosepalus*

Canchalagua (Tlanchalagua), Centaury, *Centaurium sp.*

Canela, Cinnamon, *Cinnamomum sp.*

Cañutillo (Popotillo), Mormon Tea, *Ephedra sp.*

Cañutillo Del Llano (Cora de Caballo), Horsetail,
    Equisetum arvense

Cebolla, Onion, *Allium cepa*

Cedro (Sabinus Macho), Cedar, *Juniperus sp.,*
    Juniperus scopularum, J. communis

Chamiso Hediondo, Sagebrush (New Mexico), Taos Sage,
    Artemisia tridentata

Chuchupate (Oshá), Mountain Ginseng, Colorado Coughroot,
    Ligusticum porteri

Cilantro, Coriander, *Coriandrum sativum*

Clavel (Encarnación), Carnation, *Dianthus caryophyllus*

Clavo, Cloves, *Caryophyllos aromaticus*

Coco, Coconut, *Cocos nucifera*

Cola de Caballo (Cañutillo Del Llano), Horsetail,
  Equisetum arvense
Comino, Cumin, *Cuminum cyminum*
Consuelda (Sinfito), Comfrey, *Symphitum officinalis*
Corteza de Mora, Mulberry, *Morus nigra, M. alba*
Cota, Indian/Hopi/Navajo Tea, *Thelesperma megapotamicum,*
  T. gracile
Cuachalalate, Juliana, *Amphipterygium adstringens*
Cucurbita (Pepo, Pimentón), Cayenne Pepper (Red Pepper),
  Capsicum frutescens
Damiana de California, Damian, *Turnera diffusa*
Delfinio (Espuela de Caballero), Delphinium (Larkspur),
  Delphinium sp.
Diente de León, Dandelion, *Taraxacum officinale*
Doradilla, Resurrection Plant, *Selaginella pilifera*
Encarnación (Clavel), Carnation, *Dianthus caryophyllus*
Encino, Oak, *Quercus sp.*
Enebro (Tascate), Juniper, *Juniperis communis*
Enotera (Flor de San Juan), Evening Primrose, *Oenothera sp.*
Epazote, Mexican Tea (Wormseed), *Chenopodium ambrosioides*
Espliego (Lavanda, Alhucema), Lavender, *Lavandula sp.*
Espuela de Caballero (Delfinio), Delphinium (Larkspur),
  Delphinium sp.
Estafiate, Mugwort (Western), *Artemisia ludoviciana*
Estramonio (Toalache, Floripondio), Jimson Weed (Loco Weed),
  Datura stramonium
Eucalypto, Eucalyptus, *Eucalyptus sp.*
Flor de Azahar, Citron Flower, *Citrus sp.*
Flor de Corazón (Magnolia), Magnolia, *Talauma mexicana*
Flor de Tila, Linden Flower, *Tilla sp.*
Flor de Manita, Handflower, *Chiranthodendron pentadactylon*
Flor de San Juan (Enotera), Evening Primrose, *Oenothera sp.*

Flores de Belin, Lady Slipper, *Cypripedium sp.*

Floripondio (Estramonio, Toalache), Jimson Weed (Loco Weed),
Datura stramonium

Fresno, Ash, *Fraxinus sp.*

Geranio (Patita de Leon), Geranium (Wild),
Geranium caespitosum

Girasol, Sunflower, *Helianthus annuus*

Gobernadora (Hediondilla), Creosote Bush, *Larrea tridentata*

Gordolobo (Punchon), Mullein (Great Mullein),
Verbascum thapsus

Grano de Lino (Linaza), Flax, *Linum usitatissimum*

Guayabo, Guava, *Psidium guajava*

Hamula (Prodigiosa), Bricklebush, *Brickellia sp.*

Hediondilla (Gobernadora), Creosote Bush, *Larrea tridentata*

Hierba Buena (Yerba Buena, Menta), Mint, *Mentha spicata*
(Spearmint), *Menta piperata* (Peppermint)

Hierba de Buey (Tripa de Judas, Tumbavaquero), Morning
Glory, *Ipomoea stans*

Hierba del Soldado (Tapacola, Salvia de Monte), Tapacola,
Waltheria americana

Higuera, Fig, *Ficus carica*

Higuerilla (Palma Christi), Castor Bean, *Ricinus communis*

Hinojo, Fennel, *Foeniculum vulgare*

Hojas de Callito (Linaria), Toadflax, *Linaria vulgaris*

Huisache, Huisache, *Acacia sp.*

Inmortal, Antelope Horns, *Asclepias asperula*

Jara (Jarita, Sáuce, Sáuz), Willow (esp. White Willow), *Salix sp.*

Jarita (Jara, Sáuce, Sáuz), Willow (esp. White Willow), *Salix sp.*

Jengibre (Ajenjibre), Ginger, *Zingiber officinale*

Jicama (Xiquima), Yam Bean, *Pachyrhizus erosus*

Jiguilete (Añil), Indigo, *Indigofera anil, Indigofera sp.*

La Chaya, Tree Spinach, *Cnidoscolus chayamansa*

Laurel, Bay, *Laurus nobilis*

Lavanda (Alhucema, Espliego), Lavender, *Lavandula sp.*

Lechuga, Lettuce, *Lactuca sativa*

Limón, Lemon, *Citrus limon*

Linaria (Hojas de Callito), Toadflax, *Linaria vulgaris*

Linaza (Grano de Lino), Flax, *Linum usitatissimum*

Lirio de Los Valles, Lily of the Valley, *Convallaria magalis*

Magnolia (Flor de Corazón), Magnolia, *Talauma mexicana*

Maguey (Agave), Century Plant, Mescal, *Agave sp.*

Mal Mujer (Ortiga Mayor), Nettle (Stinging Nettle), *Urtica sp.*

Malva, Mallow, *Malva neglecta*

Malva, Musk Mallow, *Malva sp.*

Manzanilla, Chamomile, *Matricaria recutita (German)*,
   M. nobile (Roman), M. chamomile (American Southwest)

Manzanitas (Pingüica, Tepezcuite), Bearberry,
   Arctostaphylos uva-ursi

Marijuana, Marijuana, *Cannabis sativa*

Mariquilla, Goldenrod, *Solidago sp.*

Marrubio Concha, Horehound, *Marrubium vulgare*

Matarique, Matarique, *Cacalia decomposita*

Mejorana, Marjoram (Sweet Marjoram), *Origanum majorana*

Menta (Hierba Buena, Yerba Buena), Mint, *Mentha spicata*
   (Spearmint), *Mentha piperata* (Peppermint)

Mesquite, Mesquite, *Prosopis julifera*

Milenrama (Plumajillo), Yarrow, *Achillea lanulosa*

Moja de Guaco (Aristoloquia), Birthwort, *Aristolochia clematitis*,
   A. serpentaria, A. tomentosa, Aristolochia sp.

Mostaza, Mustard, *Brassica nigra, Sinapis alba*

Naranja, Orange (Seville Orange), *Citrus aurantium*

Naranja Agria, Bitter Orange, *Citrus aurantium*

Nogal, Walnut, *Juglans regia, J. Major*

Nopal, Prickly Pear Cactus, *Opuntia sp.*

Nuez (Pacanero), Pecan, *Carya illinoinensis*
Nuez Moscada, Nutmeg, *Myristica fragrans*
Ocotillo, Candlewood, *Fouqueria splendens*
Olivo, Olive, *Olea europea*
Olmo, Elm, *Ulmus sp.*
Oregano, Oregano (Wild Marjoram), *Monarda sp.*
Ortiga Mayor (Mal Mujer), Nettle (Stinging Nettle), *Urtica sp.*
Oshá (Chuchupate), Mountain Ginseng, Colorado Coughroot,
  Ligusticum porteri
Pacanero (Nuez), Pecan, *Carya illinoinensis*
Palma Christi (Higuerilla), Castor Bean, *Ricinus communis*
Palo Amargo, Mexican Quinine, *Hintonia latiflora*
Papa, Potato, *Solanum tuberosum*
Papaya, Papaya, *Carica papaya*
Passiflora (Passionaria), Passion Flower, *Passiflora sp.*
Passionaria (Passiflora), Passion Flower, *Passiflora sp.*
Patita de Leon (Geranio), Geranium (Wild),
  Geranium caespitosum
Pelos de Elote (Barbas de Elote), Cornsilk, *Zea mays*
Pepo (Cucurbita, Pimentón), Cayenne Pepper (Red Pepper),
  Capsicum frutescens
Pericón (Yerba Anís, Santa Maria), Marigold (Sweet),
  Tagetes lucida
Perejil, Parsley, *Petroselinum crispum*
Pimentón (Cucurbita, Pepo), Cayenne Pepper (Red Pepper),
  Capsicum frutescens
Pingüica (Tepezcuite, Manzanitas), Bearberry,
  Arctostaphylos uva-ursi
Pino, Pine, *Pinus sp.*
Piñon (Trementina de Piñon), Pinyon, *Pinus edulis*
Pirú (Pirul), Pepper Tree, *Schinus molle*

Pirul (Pirú), Pepper Tree, *Schinus molle*

Plumajillo (Milenrama), Yarrow, *Achillea lanulosa*

Poleo, Brook Mint, *Mentha arvenis*

Poleo de Casa (Poleo de Chino), Pennyroyal,
   Hedeoma oblongifolium (commercial plant: *H. pulegoides)*

Poleo de Chino (Poleo de Casa), Pennyroyal,
   Hedeoma oblongifolium (commercial plant: *H. pulegoides)*

Ponil, Apache Plume, *Falugia paradoxa*

Popotillo (Cañutillo), Mormon Tea, *Ephedra sp.*

Prodigiosa (Hamula), Bricklebush, *Brickellia sp.*

Punchon (Gordolobo), Mullein (Great Mullein),
   Verbascum thapsus

Raiz de Cocolmeca (Zarzaparilla), Sarsaparilla, *Smilax sp.*

Raiz de Valeriana, Valerian, *Valeriana sp.*

Romero, Rosemary, *Rosmarinus officinalis*

Rosa de Castilla, Rose of Castille, *Rosa sp.*, possibly *R. centifolia*

Ruda, Rue, *Ruda sp.*

Sabila, Aloe Vera, *Aloe barbadensis, Aloe vera*

Sabinus Macho (Cedro), Cedar, *Juniperus sp.*,
   Juniperus scopularum, J. communis

Salvia, Sage, *Salvia hispanica* or *tilliaefolia, Salvia sp.*

Salvia de Monte (Hierba del Soldado, Tapacola), Tapacola,
   Waltheria americana

Santa Maria (Altimisa Mexicana), Feverfew,
   Chrysanthemum parthenium

Santa Maria (Pericón, Yerba Anís), Marigold (Sweet),
   Tagetes lucida

Sáuce (Jarita, Jara, Sáuz), Willow (esp. White Willow), *Salix sp.*

Saúco, Elder Flower, *Sambucus nigra, S. Canadensis*

Sáuz (Sáuce, Jarita, Jara), Willow (esp. White Willow), *Salix sp.*

Siempreviva, Houseleek, *Sedum sp.*

Sinfito (Consuelda), Comfrey, *Symphitum officinalis*

Tapacola (Salvia de Monte, Hierba del Soldado), Tapacola, *Waltheria americana*

Tascate (Enebro), Juniper, *Juniperis communis*

Té de Limón (Zacate de Limón), Lemon Grass, *Cymbopogon citratus*

Tepezcohuite, Tepezcohuite, *Mimosa tenuiflora*

Tepezcuite (Manzanitas, Pingüica), Bearberry, *Arctostaphylos uva-ursi*

Tlanchalagua (Canchalagua), Centaury, *Centaurium sp.*

Tlanchichinole, Tree Gloxina, *Kohleria deppeana*

Toalache (Floripondio, Estramonio), Jimson Weed (Loco Weed), *Datura stramonium*

Tomillo, Thyme, *Thymus vulgaris*

Toronjil, Lemon Balm (Giant Hyssop), *Cedronella mexicana*, *Melissa sp.*

Trementina de Piñon (Piñon), Pinyon, *Pinus edulis*

Tripa de Judas (Hierba de Buey, Tumbavaquero), Morning Glory, *Ipomoea stans*

Tronadora, Trumpet Flower (Yellowbells), *Tecoma stans*

Tumbavaquero (Hierba de Buey, Tripa de Judas), Morning Glory, *Ipomoea stans*

Uña de Gato, Cat's Claw, *Uncaria tomentosa*

Vainilla, Vanilla, *Vanilla plantifolia* or *Vanilla fragrans*

Verbena, Vervain, *Verbena sp.*

Violeta, Violet, *Viola sp.*

Xiquima (Jicama), Yam Bean, *Pachyrhizus erosus*

Yerba Buena (Hierba Buena, Menta), Mint, *Mentha spicata* (Spearmint), *Mentha piperata* (Peppermint)

Yerba Anís (Santa Maria, Pericón), Marigold (Sweet), *Tagetes lucida*

Yerba de la Negrita, Scarlet Globemallow, *Sphaeralcea coccinea*

Yerba del Sapo, Sea Holly (Snake Buttonroot), *Eryngium sp.*

Yerba Mansa, Swamp Root, *Anemopsis californica*

Yerba Santa, Mountain Balm (Holly Herb),
   Eriodictyon angustifolia, E. californicum

Zabila, Aloe Vera, *Aloe barbadensis, Aloe vera*

Zacate de Limón (Té de Limón), Lemon Grass,
   Cymbopogon citratus

Zarzamora, Blackberry, *Rubus strigosus*

Zarzaparilla (Raiz de Cocolmeca), Sarsaparilla, *Smilax sp.*

Zitsim (Altimisa, Zizim), Mugwort (Mountain Mugwort),
   Artemisia franserioides

Zizim (Altimisa, Zitzim), Mugwort (Mountain Mugwort),
   Artemisia franserioides

Glossary of Herbs

Names of plants and herbs listed below are generally, although not always, listed in the following order: a common name first (often English, but sometimes a Spanish or even an indigenous name), followed by a common Spanish name (or a second Spanish name), followed by the botanical, or Latin, name. In some cases, a plant name such as *hierba buena* (or yerba buena) applies to many different plants; in this case, I settled on what appeared to be the most widespread application of the term yerba buena that I could discern, which is peppermint and spearmint. In some cases, one Spanish (or indigenous) term is given and then another common Spanish term is given (or sometimes only one Spanish name is given), where there is no commonly used English name.

In all cases, I have tried to include a specific botanical name, but sometimes, alas, the identification of the plant is so vague in the tradition and the literature that I have indicated this vagueness in the botanical name—e.g., pine, where a wide variety of different pine species could be substituted interchangeably, I have indicated this by the suffix "sp." rather than naming a specific species. Hence,

Pinus sp. indicates pine of indeterminate species as opposed to, say, *Pinus ponderosa*, ponderosa pine. For those who prefer to reference plants by their Spanish names, an alphabetical listing has been provided in the appendix.

Aloe Vera || *Zabila, Sabila* || *Aloe barbadensis, Aloe vera*

The healing properties of aloe vera have been known for centuries—in fact, the first reference to it was made in 333 BC. Aloe vera, part of the same family as onion and garlic (not of cactus as is widely supposed because of the plant's spines), grows where there is no danger of freezing. In the United States, this means South Texas or Florida. Of course, aloe vera can also be cultivated as a houseplant.

Because aloe vera has become very popular, it is possible to buy the extracted gel in bottles for use on cuts, burns, rashes, insect bites, acne, or as a wrinkle preventative. This gel is usually liquefied and often is stabilized so that it needs no refrigeration. Mexican-Americans mix the gel with water and drink it to treat arthritis, rheumatism, and stomach disorders. If you are using the plant itself rather than the bottled gel, simply break off a leaf, slit it, squeeze out the gel that you find inside, and apply. Aloe vera can also be used as a meat tenderizer.

Aniseed || *Anís, Yerba Anís, Pericón* || *Pimpinella anisum*

Use for muscle pain in chest and shoulders, when ground and mixed with whiskey and rubbed on affected areas. When ground and drunk with hot water, can be used to alleviate symptoms of pneumonia. Take as tea for stomach problems, coughing, and colic. See Mexican Tarragon.

Antelope Horns || *Inmortal* || *Asclepias asperula*

Inmortal is used for respiratory ailments since it stimulates the lungs and expels phlegm. Do not use during pregnancy, but can be used to expel afterbirth.

Apache Plume || *Ponil* || *Fallugia paradoxa*

The roots and flower tops of *ponil* are used as a hair rinse to strengthen the hair. The tea can be taken as a remedy for coughs.

Arnica || *Arnica* || *Arnica cardifolia*

Arnica is used in tincture form externally for arthritis and sprains.

Arnica Mexicana (Camphor Weed) || *Arnica Mexicana* || *Heterotheca sp.*

Arnica Mexicana is used in solution form for stomach discomforts such as gas and cramps and also as a skin wash for minor dermatological disorders.

Ash || *Fresno* || *Fraxinus sp.*

Ash is said to be a snake repellent, so effective that some people, when venturing into snake-infested areas, carried boughs of it with them. This rumor may have grown as the result of mention in a 1597 book titled *Gerard's Herbal*, to wit: "serpents dare not be so bolde as to touch the morning and evening shadows of the (Ash) tree." In any case, ash is said to be a remedy for snake bite (should carrying these boughs fail to ward the snakes away). To use in this manner, make a strong tea from the leaves and drink it if you are bitten. This tea is also supposedly a remedy for gout and rheumatism and can be taken to reduce fever. Ash is also said to have the ability to increase longevity, and, when used for this purpose, should be ingested each day. Ash is also rumored to be an aphrodisiac.

Basil (Sweet Basil) || *Albahaca* || *Ocimum basilicum*

Basil is an easy herb to grow. Its leaves and sometimes the flowering tips of the plant are used, either fresh or dried, to make a tea. This tea is supposed to have sedative and antispasmodic properties and therefore is often administered to those suffering from susto or shock. In a more concentrated form, basil tea can be used as a gargle for sore throat or to heal sores in the mouth. The same tea can also be used externally on insect stings. A decoction of basil, honey, and nutmeg is supposedly good to give to a mother immediately after childbirth to aid in expelling the afterbirth.

Bay || *Laurel* || *Laurus nobilis*
Bay is a tree whose leaves are used to make a tea that is said to cure colic and diarrhea. Bay leaves are supposed to keep insects away and are often tucked into the band of a hat for this purpose. The oil from the berries can be extracted, too, and applied externally to muscles that are sore because of rheumatism or overexertion.

Bayberry || *Arbol de la Cera* || *Myrica californica, M. cerifera*
Swallowing a nickel-sized piece of the berry wax or chewing the dry berries will, it is said, quiet a cough or cure dysentery. A teaspoon of the liquid extracted from either the root or the bark has a similar use. It will supposedly ward off a cold if it is taken at the very first sign of the cold's onset. Still another method of treating or preventing a cold is to dry a piece of the root bark and powder it, then make a tea of the powder. The same powder can be used as a snuff to cure nasal congestion. Or the powder can be mixed with water to make an astringent mouthwash, especially good as a remedy for sore or bleeding gums.

Bearberry, Uva Ursi || *Pingüica, Tepezcuite, Manzanitas* || *Arctostaphylos uva-ursi*
A cold tea is made from the leaves and drunk for urethral and bladder infections. Cascara sagrada (sacred bark, *Rhamnus purshiana*) is also called bearberry but is used as a laxative.

Birthwort || *Moja de Guaco, Aristoloquia* || *Aristolochia clematitis, A. serpentaria, A. tomentosa, Aristolochia sp.*

A tea made from birthwort causes sweating (that is, it is a diaphoretic) and, reportedly, is a stimulant. Large doses of this tea, however, can cause vomiting and stomach pains. Birthwort is also used in the form of a tincture, which means that its leaves are soaked in alcohol, then strained out and the resulting liquid saved to be applied as an antiseptic in cases of insect bite, especially if the insects are poisonous. There are many different kinds of birthwort, and one must take care in choosing the variety and dosage for one's particular need.

Blackberry || *Zarzamora* || *Rubus strigosus*

The leaves are boiled for about ten minutes and the resulting liquid is used to rinse out the mouth if the gums are inflamed or if ulcers are present in the mouth. The same decoction, in lesser strength, is taken for diarrhea. The root bark is more potent than the leaves and is also used.

Borage || *Borraja* || *Borago officinalis*

This herb was known by the Moors as abou-rach, "the father of sweat." Indeed, borage is said to purify the body by increasing not only sweat but urine as well. Drinking a tea made of borage is also alleged to keep the body cool, so it is sometimes used as a summer drink. It is also offered to those suffering from fever for the same cooling effect. Borage tea is considered especially effective when the fever is attributable to measles.

Because borage increases the flow of urine, it is sometimes used to treat bladder infections. Scientific analysis of borage shows that it contains potassium.

Bougainvillea || *Bugambilia, Buganvilla* || *Bougainvillea spectabilis*
A tea can be made from the flowers and used to combat a cough or sore throat. Combined with mullein, gordolobo, eucalyptus leaves, and honey, can be used to treat bronchitis; this combination of herbs is prepared by an infusion (soaked in water).

Bricklebush || *Hamula, Prodigiosa* || *Brickellia sp.*
Used in tea form to control Type II diabetes. Also used for constipation and stomach ailments caused by bile and gallbladder stones.

Brook Mint || *Poleo* || *Mentha arvensis*
Poleo settles the stomach, relieves stomach discomfort such as nausea and diarrhea, reduces fevers, and helps alleviate headache pain. This plant can be infused and sweetened, or the steam inhaled. When infused and sweetened with honey, it is used for a hoarse and raspy throat. See Pennyroyal.

Cactus—see Prickly Pear Cactus.

Camomile—see Chamomile.

Camphor || *Alcanfor* || *Cinnamomum camphora*
The oil from the leaves of this tree is used as an anaphrodisiac, that is, a substance that diminishes sexual desire. This oil is obtained through an elaborate process of steaming the branches, pressing the liquid produced into crystals, and then liquefying the crystals. The oil, then, is best purchased. Camphor is most often used to treat earache and as a rub on rheumatic joints or on the forehead in the case of headache.

Carnation || *Clavel, Encarnación* || *Dianthus caryophyllus*
Soak fresh flower petals in water, adding sugar to thicken into a syrup. When strained, this syrup is used to combat indigestion, gas, and bloating due to overeating. It is also used for cough.

Castor Bean || *Higuerilla, Palma Christi* || *Ricinus communis*
All parts of this plant, including the bean, which is the seed of the plant, are poisonous. Oil is extracted from the bean by pressing it, however, and serves as an excellent remedy for irritations of the gastrointestinal tract and the genitourinary system. All herbals advise that one never under any circumstances consume the seed. It would probably be best to purchase castor oil if one wishes to use it. In parts of Mexico, the leaves are used as a poultice for swollen joints and bruises.

Cat's Claw || *Uña de Gato* || *Uncaria tomentosa*
The Peruvian variety is the kind that you want, not the American (*Acacia greggii*, which is used externally for muscle pain). Native Ashanica Indians used it to treat a wide range of health problems associated with the immune and digestive systems. The plant is also taken as a general disease preventative.

Cayenne Pepper (Red Pepper) || *Cucurbita, Pepo, Pimentón* ||
Capsicum frutescens
A pinch of powdered peppers in drinking water will ward off susto or shock. Cayenne can be applied directly to razor cuts as a styptic, e.g., a substance that stops bleeding. Cayenne pepper can also be brewed as a tea and consumed in cold weather, it is said, to keep the body warm. It is also shaken into shoes to keep the feet from getting cold.

Cedar || *Sabinus Macho, Cedro* || *Juniperus sp.,*
Juniperus scopularum, J. communis
A tea made from cedar is used in cases of malaria. Cedar, however,

is also used in the rituals of curanderismo. In cases of susto, or magical fright, the afflicted person is swept with branches of the cedar tree while the curandero recites the Apostles' Creed.

As with other widely applied tree and plant names, cedar seems to be used to describe a range of evergreen trees and shrubs. In the Southwest, *J. communis* seems to be one of the trees identified as having medicinal properties (Spanish name *sabinus macho*). In the case of this Southwestern juniper, the tea is used for urinary tract infections and for fever reduction.

Centaury || *Tlanchalagua, Canchalagua* || *Centaurium sp.*
Combined with other plants, it is taken before meals to help induce weight loss.

Century Plant (Mescal) || *Maguey, Agave* || *Agave sp.*
This plant is a modern source of steroids. Some maguey plants contain a substance similar to cortisone. The plant looks a great deal like aloe vera, though it does not have the spines. It is applied to wounds in a similar way. Occasionally the leaves are heated and used to induce draining of abscesses.

Chamomile || *Manzanilla* || *Matricaria recutita (German),*
M. nobile (Roman), M. chamomilia (American Southwest)
Chamomile is a member of the thistle family. Its flowers as well as its leaves are used to make a tea that is taken to calm the nerves and to aid digestion. A stronger tea is consumed when fever is present. Because chamomile has, despite its sweet odor, a bitter taste, it is often sweetened with honey and flavored with lemon. Chamomile tea, without additives, can be used externally as an eyewash. The steam from boiling chamomile is also used to clear the nasal passages from congestion. A tent is made by covering the head with a towel and letting the ends hang down over a pot of boiling water

with chamomile in it. The vapor that is trapped in the tent is then inhaled. This procedure is also said to cleanse pores and is sometimes recommended as a beauty treatment. Furthermore, when this decoction is cool, it supposedly makes a good after-shampoo rinse!

It is said, too, that those who wish to break the nicotine habit should chew fresh or dried chamomile flowers when the urge for a cigarette strikes.

Cinnamon || *Canela* || *Cinnamomum sp.*
An oil is released by bruising the bark, leaves, fruit, or root of the cinnamon plant. This oil can be used as a rub on rheumatic aches. More commonly, strips of cinnamon bark can be grated or bruised and then used to make a tea that is taken to aid digestion or stimulate the appetite. Cinnamon is also available in powdered form and can be used alone as a tea or to flavor other teas. Much lore surrounds cinnamon, which reportedly was used in Egypt for embalming and in witchcraft. As a remnant of the latter, cinnamon is said to be used as incense in order to increase the sexual desire of women.

Citron Flowers || *Flor de Azahar* || *Citrus sp.*
The flowers from the orange or lemon tree can be picked fresh and brewed as a tea to cure insomnia.

Cloves || *Clavo* || *Caryophyllus aromamaticus*
One can chew a clove to kill the pain of a toothache or wrap it in cotton and place it in the ear to treat an earache. Oil of cloves can be rubbed on the gums to relieve pain, too. Cloves, when chewed, are said to be an aphrodisiac. A few drops of oil of cloves in water is taken as an antiemetic, e.g., to stop vomiting.

Coconut || *Coco* || *Cocos nucifera*
Coconut water is taken in the morning for several days to rid the stomach of amoebae.

Comfrey || *Sinfito, Consuelda* || *Symphitum officinalis*
The root and foliage of this plant contain a cell proliferant, and this is why the plant is commonly used to heal wounds. Comfrey, in fact, is considered the best of all healing herbs.

It is used in a number of ways. A decoction of comfrey leaves is used as a disinfectant to bathe wounds and sores. Or, a maceration of leaves and roots can be applied either to heal a wound or to stop bleeding. Comfrey compresses will reportedly take the sting out of bites and burns, reduce swelling, and promote healing. While comfrey is mostly used externally, one can drink the water in which the roots have been soaked, presumably to stop internal bleeding or to slow the menstrual flow when it seems too profuse.

Coriander || *Cilantro* || *Coriandrum sativum*
A tea made from the dried seeds is taken to cure nausea and diarrhea. Coriander is also used as an anaphrodisiac.

Cornsilk || *Barbas de Elote, Pelos de Elote* || *Zea mays*
According to herbalists, the Cornsilk strands should be boiled and the resulting liquid drunk to treat bladder and kidney ailments. Cornsilk is said to relieve water retention and thus is given in the morning to children who wet the bed. This is rumored to "drain" them during the day and thus keep them dry at night. When used as a bedwetting remedy, cornsilk is sometimes mixed with agrimony (*Agrimonia gryposepala*). It also is supposed to relieve the painful urination sometimes associated with prostate problems.

Cota—see Indian/Hopi/Navajo Tea.

Creosote Bush (Chaparral) || *Gobernadora, Hediondilla* ||
Larrea tridentata
Taken as a tea made from the leaves of the plant, creosote bush is
though to relieve kidney problems. More widely, the leaves are
powdered and applied externally to disinfect wounds.

Cuachalalate (Juliana) || *Cuachalalate* ||
Amphipterygium adstringens
The bark is boiled and used for vaginal washes, to clean ulcers and
chronic wounds.

Cudweed—see Mullein.

Cumin || *Comino* || *Cuminum cyminum*
This plant's seeds are boiled to make a mild and soothing tea for
teething babies.

Damian || *Damiana de California* || *Turnera diffusa*
This plant is used as an aphrodisiac, as a tonic, and to soothe internal inflammations.

Dandelion || *Diente de León* || *Taraxacum officinale*
This humble and common plant has many medicinal uses. A
decoction made of the whole plant is said to be a good liniment,
while a tea made of the leaves and roots alone will act as a
diuretic, thus cleansing the body of impurities. In this latter
capacity, dandelion tea is often used as a restorative after hepatitis. In high doses, dandelion tea is said to dissolve kidney and
bladder stones. It is also allegedly an antipyretic, e.g., used to
reduce fever. When the roots alone are ground and boiled, the

resulting mixture is reputedly a laxative that aids the function of the liver.

But Dandelion has a myriad of external uses, too. The juice squeezed from any part of the plant, for instance, is applied to warts. A handful of the flowers boiled in water for half an hour and strained is said to make an excellent toilet water.

Delphinium (Larkspur) || *Espuela de Caballero, Delfinio* || *Delphinium sp.*

The flowers and seeds are ground and soaked in either alcohol or vinegar. This mixture has been used externally to attack body lice, particularly pubic lice. It should be applied after a hot bath for four or five days in a row. It does not always kill the eggs, so the person using it should keep an eye out for reinfestation. It also can be used on pets.

Elder Flower || *Saúco* || *Sambucus nigra, S. canadensis*

The flowers are the mildest and safest part of the plant and inhaling the steam as the flowers are boiling is said to be good for the skin, as is applying the water in which elder flowers have soaked overnight. A tea made from the bark is diuretic and a laxative, and thus is said to be good to consume in cases of water retention. The same tea promotes sweating and is often given to those with fever. Fresh elder leaves, crushed and mixed with olive oil, can be applied to hemorrhoids for relief. The blue elderberries can be eaten, but the red are toxic.

Elm || *Olmo* | *Ulmus sp.*

Herbalists advise that the inner bark be dried, then soaked in cold water, then brought to a boil for ten minutes. The resulting fluid can be drunk to relieve edema, or swelling due to water retention. This elm mixture has also reportedly been taken to clear the complexion. The liquid can also be used externally to soak compresses that are then applied to skin eruptions.

Eucalyptus || *Eucalipto* || *Eucalyptus sp.*
The leaves are used as a tea to promote digestion, but more often they are boiled and the steam inhaled to relieve congestion and cough. Asthma sufferers can smoke dried eucalyptus leaves for relief.

Evening Primrose || *Flor de San Juan, Enotera* || *Oenothera sp.*
The oil from the flowers, according to an article in *Redbook* magazine, can be taken to combat the battery of symptoms known as "premenstrual syndrome," e.g., bloating, irritability, and headache. The same article reported that evening primrose oil had been touted in the early 1700s as "The King's Cure All."

Evening primrose oil has also been used to treat eczema and British studies have shown a reduction in the scaly, itchy skin eruptions associated with that disease. It is also being tested as a treatment for alcoholism. The active ingredient in evening primrose oil is a chemical called gamma-linolenic acid.

Fennel || *Hinojo* || *Foeniculum vulgare*
The leaves, seeds, steams and roots are used to make a tea said to stimulate appetite, soothe stomachaches and colic, and act as a diuretic. Dry fennel seeds, too, when cooked in a cupful of milk and drunk as hot as possible, are said to eliminate gas. The same mixture is supposed to be soothing to flu sufferers, too. The seeds boiled in water are said to give off steam that is inhaled for migraine headache relief. In addition, fennel is thought to have magical powers. Sprigs of it are still hung about the home to rid it of evil spirits.

Feverfew || *Santa Maria, Altamisa Mexicana* ||
Chrysanthemum parthenium
For colds, flu, and fever. Also used to induce menstruation. One source warns strongly against using this herb during pregnancy.

Fig || *Higuera* || *Ficus carica*

Cooked figs are eaten as a laxative and to cure sore throat and cough. The figs are also given to children with scarlet fever or chicken pox. Externally, a cooked fig can be split open and applied hot to sores and boils. In addition, the milky sap, which issues from the snapped branch of a fig tree, can be applied to corns and warts in order to dissolve them.

Flax || *Grano de Lino, Linaza* || *Linum usitatissimum*

Flaxseed, also called linseed, is boiled in water to make a disinfectant useful for bathing sores and rinsing out the mouth. Flaxseed is also said to be useful as a poultice or plaster, which is applied to boils, abscesses, or even tumors. Modern herbals caution not to use boiled linseed oil from the hardware store!

Garden Heliotrope—see Valerian.

Garlic || *Ajo* || *Allium sativum*

This is another revered medicinal plant, and it is said to cure a multiplicity of ills. It should be used fresh, as it loses its potency when processed into powder. When a clove of garlic is crushed and mixed with olive oil, for instance, it serves as an unguent to be used on burns and abrasions. A clove peeled and wrapped in gauze can be inserted into the ear to cure earache. And three to four peeled cloves soaked in a pint of brandy that has been kept in a dark place, say, a closet, for about fourteen days will, when strained, serve as an effective cough syrup for asthma sufferers and those troubled by coughing spells.

The efficacy of garlic has been studied and various surprising facts about it have emerged. One German study, for example, says that garlic helps to break up cholesterol in the blood vessels, thereby reducing the risk of heart attack. A Japanese study claims that garlic rids the system of various poisons such as lead or mercury. A Russian study is said to have shown that application of a garlic preparation retarded tumor growth. There have been studies (such as one reported in *Science* magazine in 1957) where cancer-ridden mice that ate garlic were observed to live longer than those who did not eat it.

There is no question that garlic has antibacterial and anti-inflammatory properties. For years, it has been mashed and mixed with honey or milk or softened bread and then applied to wounds—even scorpion bites!

Garlic is also made into a tea that is used to treat stomach ulcers as well as liver and kidney disorders. One herbal advises that three cloves eaten and washed down with a glass of milk will prevent tuberculosis.

Two additional practices involve crushing garlic and mixing it with brown sugar to use as a cough syrup in cases of whooping cough and the practice of eating garlic cloves whole to prevent scurvy. Another external use is to mash garlic cloves into a paste and, using honey to bind the cloves, apply it to the scalp to cure dandruff.

Gayfeather, Blazing Star || *Cachana* || *Liatris punctado*
The roots are used to protect against mal de ojo, or evil eye. The smoke from the fuzzy roots is inhaled for nosebleeds and tonsillitis.

Geranium (Wild) || *Geranio, Patita de Leon* || *Geranium caespitosum*
A tea made from the leaves is a good aromatic body wash. This tea is high in calcium and is often taken as a dietary supplement. It is also used as a gargle for sore throat.

Ginger || *Ajenjibre, Jengibre* || *Zingiber officinale*
The leaves as well as the root of this plant can be used both externally and internally. Made into a tea, ginger relieves the achy feeling

often associated with the onset of flu. The same tea will reportedly relieve nausea, too. Ginger is also thought by some to be an aphrodisiac. Water with powdered ginger in it is said to be an excellent foot soak.

Goldenrod || *Mariquilla* || *Solidago sp.*
Dried and powdered leaves as well as the flowering tips of this plant make a tea that is said to combat arthritis and aid those with diabetes. Goldenrod tea is also rumored to be an effective diuretic and is used to reduce water retention and even to break up kidney stones.

Guava || *Guayabo* || *Psidium guajava*
The Aztecs used guava extract externally, as an astringent. It is also listed in some herbals as an anthelmintic, meaning that it is used to destroy intestinal worms.

Handflower || *Flor de Manita* || *Chiranthodendron pentadactylon*
This plant is combined with other plants in order to treat heart disorders.

Hierba Buena (Yerba Buena)—see Mint.

Horehound || *Marrubio Concha* || *Marrubium vulgare*
A renowned expectorant, a bitter tea is made from horehound by pouring boiling water over a handful of the leaves of the plant. This is allowed to stand for ten minutes, and the resulting fluid, when consumed, is said to stimulate menstruation, aid digestion, and reduce fever. Honey and lemon are the recommended sweetening agents. Years ago in England a beer was made from horehound. In large doses, horehound tea is used to expel intestinal worms.

**Horsetail || *Cola de Caballo, Cañutillo Del Llano* ||
*Equisetum arvense***

A concentrated decoction of this plant is useful as a lotion for washing sores and abscesses, but it can also be used to keep the feet from sweating. It contains acotanic acid, which stops secretions, thus it is thought to stop internal bleeding when made into a tea and consumed. It is taken in this way when menstruation is too profuse or when the bladder or intestines are inflamed. Horsetail is frequently used to remedy incontinence, kidney stones, and prostate gland ailments.

Houseleek (Stonecrop) || *Siempreviva* || *Sedum sp.*

The leaves can be plucked from this plant and eaten to soothe intestinal irritation, but, more often, the juice from the plant's leaves is used externally, either in a poultice or rubbed directly on sores, burns, warts, or stings. Cold houseleek poultices are applied to the head to cure headache and hot houseleek poultices are used to relive the pain and itching of hemorrhoids. The fresh leaf of a houseleek, it is said, will arrest bleeding when applied directly to a wound.

Huisache || *Huisache* || *Acacia sp.*

The leaves and bark are commonly brewed as a tea when a diuretic is needed. The same mixture can be used as a gargle for sore throat, or applied externally as an astringent.

The huisache leaves, bark, and root, when pulverized and boiled into a concentrate, are sometimes taken for cough. When brewed this way, herbalists advise that the dosage is critical.

The fresh huisache flowers, picked in the spring, can be boiled to create vapors. These are inhaled, using the method outlined earlier (see Chamomile).

**Indian/Hopi/Navajo Tea || *Cota* || *Thelesperma megapotamicum,
T. gracile***
This plant is made into a tea as a remedy for stomach disorders. It
is also known for its excellent taste as a purely recreational drink
and as a diuretic.

Indigo || *Añil, Jiguilete* || *Indigofera anil, Indigofera sp.*
A tea made from the leaves is used to treat empacho and even
epilepsy. Externally, the leaves are used as a poultice on the forehead
to relieve headache. In addition, indigo seeds can be ground and the
powder dusted over the body to destroy lice and to heal sores.

**Jimson Weed, Angel's Trumpet (Loco Weed) ||
Estramonio, Toloache, Floripondio || *Datura stramonium***
This was used as a wash on horses and cows, reportedly to keep
them from straying. Humans use the smoke from the burning
leaves of the plant to control the spasms associated with asthma.
The same smoke also dries up nasal secretions and is helpful in cases
of sinusitis. The fresh jimson weed plant makes a good poultice for
painful joints. People with hot tubs drop the leaves into the water
for this purpose (though the same can be done by soaking them in
the bathtub).

Jimson weed should never be taken internally. It can cause
coma, convulsions, and death. It is used externally only in liniments
and salves for arthritis.

Juliana—see Chuachalalate.

Juniper || *Enebro, Tascate* || *Juniperis communis*
Tea from the berries is thought to be both an aphrodisiac and a
means of birth control (a formidable combination!). More reliably,

both the leaves and berries are diuretic and used to fight water retention. The berries alone, crushed and soaked in a covered container of water, yield a liquid often used to treat cystitis and urethritis. Juniper is also used in tincture form for the same purpose. To make the tincture, macerate the berries and soak them in white wine for a week, then strain to remove all residue and keep the remaining liquid. These berries are also used to flavor gin.

Juniper berries can be used fresh or dried. They are often chewed to eliminate gas. In addition, they are often combined with the leaves and burned, both to combat bad odors and, legend says, evil influences as well. A sprig of juniper kept in a vase is said to guard the occupants of the house against evil, too.

Lady Slipper || *Flores de Belin* || *Cypripedium sp.*
Internal use is sometimes made of this plant, but this is risky since it has toxic properties. More commonly, it is used to remedy ingrown toenail. To effect this cure, mash the fresh flowers and place them on the toenail, where they should remain overnight. This procedure should be continued until the toenail grows properly.

Larkspur—see Delphinium.

Lavender || *Espliego, Alhucema, Lavanda* || *Lavandula sp.*
Internally, the flowers are brewed into a tea and taken as a sedative or an antispasmodic (the plant is classified as an antiemetic, which means it will stop vomiting). It is reputedly a cure for menstrual cramps and, as one old text puts it, "serves as a remedy for giddiness." Externally, the same tea can be used as a footbath or applied to the body as a liniment, which is said to stimulate the nerve endings. Still another external remedy that is often reported is that a few drops of essence of lavender on the forehead will cure headache and relieve depression.

But lavender has proven cosmetic uses, too. An excellent lotion can be made by mixing macerated lavender blossoms and olive oil until the mixture smells good.

Lemon || *Limón* || *Citrus limon*
Powdered bark from the root of this plant can be made into a tea and used to induce sweating and break a fever. More commonly, however, the fruit—which is certainly more readily available—is used. The juice of the lemon is known to be an antiseptic. Lemon also serves as a styptic. Half a lemon applied to a razor cut will staunch the bleeding, though the cut will sting as a result.

Lemon is rumored to cure a great many ills. For instance, legend has it that any painful spots on the body should be rubbed with half a lemon to ease the pain. To relieve a headache, an old remedy is to cut a lemon in half and apply a section to each temple. And, probably because the citric acid in lemon has a drying effect, it is used on corns and to soften rough skin spots. Of course, lemon, especially when mixed with honey, is best known as a remedy for the common cold.

Lemon Balm, Giant Hyssop || *Toronjil* || *Cedronella mexicana, Melissa sp.*
Lemon balm (Melissa) and the cedronella of Mexico are both called *toronjil*. As a tea, it is said to be effective in relieving stomach pain, gas, diarrhea, and menstrual cramps, as well as in reawakening appetite, and is also used for coping with insomnia.

Lemon Grass || *Té de Limón, Zarate de Limón* || *Cymbopogon citratus*
The tea is used to remedy stomach disorders and flatulence.

Lettuce || *Lechuga* || *Lactuca sativa*
Tea can be brewed from the leaves to relieve constipation and calm the nerves. It is often taken at bedtime to insure sound sleep. Lettuce

tea is also said to quell sexual desire. Wild lettuce is also dried and smoked for its sedative effect. The plant contains arsenic, but in small, harmless quantities.

Lily of the Valley || *Lirio de Los Valles* || *Convallaria magalis*
The dried flowers of lily of the valley were often powdered and used as a snuff. Many, however, preferred to drink an infusion of the flowers and occasionally the root. The resulting tea is said to be a cardiac tonic.

Indeed, lily of the valley acts very much like digitalis and care should be taken not to drink too much. But lily of the valley can be toxic even in small quantities. One legend says that a child died within minutes of drinking the water from a glass in which a sprig of lily of the valley had been placed!

Linden Flower || *Flor de Tila* || *Tilla sp.*
Tea made from this flower is used as a tranquilizer and is taken as a soporific to induce sleep at bedtime.

Magnolia || *Flor de Corazón, Magnolia* || *Talauma mexicana*
Those who have had heart attacks were advised by some herbalists to drink a tea made from the petals of the magnolia blossoms. Indeed, the Aztec name for magnolia was yoloxochitl, which means "heart flower." The bark of the magnolia tree, when powdered and soaked in water, has been shown to be a heart stimulant. But, in addition to this use, the Aztecs prepared a tonic with the dried blossoms to treat mental stupor and senility.

Mallow || *Malva* || *Malva neglecta*
The flowers of this plant can be softened in water and then chewed to relieve the pain of a toothache. The flowers can also be brewed by

infusion into a mouthwash that is said to soothe irritations of the mouth and gums.

The fresh or dried leaves, too, can be used, either to make a poultice or brewed to make a tea. In the latter form, mallow soothes the mucous membranes and is therefore considered a good remedy for sore throat or even sore tonsils. Some claim mallow tea will calm intestinal irritation.

Externally, mallow tea is used as a body wash, particularly on children, to reduce fever, or to clean wounds and bruises. Crushed leaves are also applied to relieve the inflammation associated with mumps. However it is used, it should be washed well because dogs tend to choose the mallow plant to mark their territory.

Marigold || *Caléndula* || *Calendula officinalis*

The whole plant can be used in tincture and applied to sores. An infusion of the fresh or dried flowers, allowed to stand for ten to fifteen minutes can, similarly, be used as a lotion. A decoction made from the root can be drunk as a tea to relieve gout and rheumatism. It is also said that applying the leaves of a marigold plant to calluses will soften them and eventually make them disappear.

Marigold (Sweet) || *Pericón, Yerba Anís, Santa Maria* || *Tagetes lucida*

This plant is used for stomachaches and fever. Hot baths with marigold are used for women in childbirth and to bathe children for a soothing and calming effect.

Marijuana || *Marijuana* || *Cannabis sativa*

In tincture, marijuana is rubbed on rheumatic limbs. Brewed as a tea, it is taken to quiet coughing spells (especially when mixed with horehound). In fact, a weak marijuana tea is given to colicky babies.

Externally, a poultice made of the leaves and roots of the plant is said to have a great deal of drawing power and therefore is applied to carbuncles and boils.

When smoked, marijuana is an intoxicant. Studies have shown, however, that smoking marijuana may be of benefit to those suffering from glaucoma as it tends to reduce ocular pressure. Because of the plant's illegality, however, it is not often used for medicinal purposes.

Marjoram (Sweet Marjoram) || *Mejorana* || *Origanum majorana*
As a tea, marjoram cures stomachache. A stronger decoction can be brewed and a cloth soaked in the mixture. This cloth is then wrapped around the throat of a person suffering from sore throat to provide relief.

Matarique || *Matarique* || *Cacalia decomposita*
A tincture from the matarique root is used for arthritis and rheumatism.

Mesquite || *Mesquite* || *Prosopis julifera*
The sap of this tree is dissolved in water and taken as a cure for dysentery. In addition, a tea infused from the seeds and bark can be consumed to combat irritations of the digestive tract. A decoction made from the leaves can be used to wash inflamed eyes.

Mexican Day Flower || *Yerba del Pollo* || *Comelina coelestis*
The entire plant is mixed with lemon juice and used as a compress to stop bleeding since it constricts the capillaries. It is used for nosebleeds, wounds, and postpartum bleeding.

Mexican Quinine || *Palo Amargo* || *Hintonia latiflora*
An infusion (plant soaked in water) is taken throughout the day to control diabetes. It is also used for liver disorders.

Mexican Tarragon || *Pericón, Santa Maria, Yerba Anís* || *Targetes sp.*

The entire plant is used for stomachaches, nausea, and colic. It is also taken for colds and fevers. See Marigold (Sweet).

Mexican Tea, Wormseed || *Epazote* || *Chenopodium ambrosioides*

Epazote is taken in small amounts as a tea to stimulate lactation for nursing mothers. This is also a popular seasoning for beans. It is used to eliminate worms in humans and animals, and to stimulate delayed menstruation. A more pungent species is *epazote de zorillo* (*chemopodium graveolens*), which is used for nervousness and depression.

Mint || *Hierba Buena, Menta, Yerba Buena* || *Mentha spicata* (Spearmint); *Mentha piperita* (Peppermint)

There are various types of easily grown mint, such as spearmint or peppermint. All are antiemetic. A tea made of any of these is said to provide relief from stomachache and nausea, but can also be taken to aid digestion. Mint tea is said to provide a mild stimulant as well, and thus is consumed to give energy and restore the spirits.

Monkshood (Wolfsbane) || *Acónito* || *Aconitum sp.*

This plant is poisonous if taken internally. The seeds, however, can be mashed and combined with lard or suet to be applied to abscesses or boils. The dried roots have been used to poison the tips of arrowheads. This plant, reportedly, is used in witchcraft.

Mormon Tea || *Cañutillo, Popotillo* || *Ephedra sp.*

This famous Southwestern plant is used for a variety of ailments. Some have even claimed it has properties that help ward off venereal diseases. Its more pedestrian uses include treating urinary tract and kidney infections as well as its use as a facial wash. *Cañutillo* is boiled and then drunk as a cold tea. It purportedly also has anti-allergenic properties.

Morning Glory || *Tumbavaquero, Hierba de Buey, Tripa de Judas* || *Ipomoea stans*

In small doses and combined with citron flowers and linden flowers, the roots are used for nervous disorders and for epileptic seizures. The roots are a remedy for spastic diarrhea, menstrual cramps, and kidney problems.

Mugwort (Mountain Mugwort) || *Altamisa, Zizim, Zitzim* || *Artemisia franserioides*

The heads of the flowers and dried leaves of this plant are used to make a tea that is said to remedy female disorders. It supposedly will combat menopausal difficulties and irregular or painful menstruation. A woman should start drinking the tea ten to twelve days before menstruation is to begin and then stop once her flow starts. Pregnant and nursing women, however, are advised to refrain from using it.

There are other uses for mugwort. An infusion of the whole plant is taken to stimulate appetite. In addition, the dried flowers are ground into a powder and used for colic as well as to rid the body of intestinal worms. The plant is also said to have magical properties and, when carried, is rumored to ward away danger. It is said that a leaf stuck in the nostril will cure a headache. Another legend advises that if one sleeps on a pillow stuffed with mugwort, one will dream of the future.

Mugwort (Western) || *Estafiate* || *Artemisia ludoviciana*

Used against flatulence, dysentery, and vomiting.

Mulberry || *Corteza de Mora* || *Morus nigra, M. alba*
The bark makes an effective mouthwash when soaked in water for twenty-four hours.

Mullein (Great Mullein) || *Gordolobo, Punchon* ||
Verbascum thapsus
This herb has been used since the middle ages. It is a noted remedy for bronchial complaints and was often fed to winded horses. Mullein has been used in various ways and to various ends. For example, smoking dried mullein leaves is said to be a remedy for the symptoms of asthma. A half-teaspoon of mullein root soaked in a quarter cup of water is supposed to cure bedwetting. The flowers of the mullein plant, soaked in hot olive oil for several hours, will, it is said, provide eardrop oil to cure an earache. The leaves and flowers—particularly the latter—are brewed in milk to make a tea for bronchial ailments. A stronger tea is said to be a sedative. In either case, when making tea, be sure to filter the coarse hairs that the flowers leave behind as these can irritate the throat. Finally, mullein can be used as a poultice for wounds, cuts, hemorrhoids, and even gout. The Spanish name gordolobo is also applied to another plant species, cudweed (*Gnaphalium sp.*).

Musk Mallow || *Malva* || *Malva sp.*
This is reportedly an antidote to snake venom and Indians in Mexico are said to wear the seeds of musk mallow in little bags around their necks when they go into a snake-infested area to work. If bitten, the poison is drawn from the wound and then the musk mallow seeds, chewed until pulpy, are placed directly over the wound. Note that musk mallow's common name in Spanish, malva, is shared with a different plant, mallow (see Mallow entry, above).

Mustard || *Mostaza* || *Brassica nigra, Sinapis alba*
The seeds are ground and mixed with lard to make a poultice to be applied wherever there is pain: the feet, the back, the chest. This allegedly cures rheumatic and arthritic pain. But mustard powder can also be mixed with water for footbaths, which are said to relieve the symptoms of colds and flu. The best-known use, however, is the plaster. To make a mustard plaster, make a paste of ground mustard seed or mustard powder, flour, and water. Wrap the paste in a damp towel or flannel cloth and rest it over the back or chest of the afflicted person. As for internal use, it is said that those who suffer from a weak stomach can strengthen it by eating mustard seeds.

Nettle (Stinging Nettle) || *Ortiga Mayor, Mal Mujer* || *Urtica sp.*
The Aztecs used this plant to reduce hemorrhaging and it is still used this way today. For example, in cases of nosebleed, a bit of moistened cotton is dipped in juice extracted by mashing the nettle plant and then placing it in the nostril. But nettle is also used internally to control excessive menstrual bleeding or even internal bleeding such as the bleeding one associates with ulcers. Nettle tea is also thought to control bedwetting, hay fever, and is used as a poultice for arthritis.

The nettle plant also has numerous other uses which have been recorded over the years. Cosmetically, the seeds can be soaked for twenty minutes in water and the water then used as a final rinse after shampooing. This will, indeed, impart a gloss to the hair. Horses used to be rubbed with the mixture to give them glossy coats. Chopped nettle leaves, too, were once fed to horses to give them more spirit. And mixed with mash, nettle supposedly enabled hens to lay more eggs. Nettle is also mentioned in some old texts as an aphrodisiac.

Nutmeg || *Nuez Moscada* || *Myristica fragrans*
The nuts are ground into a powder and boiled to produce a tea that

remedies indigestion and gas. Sometimes, too, the fleshy part of the fruit is chewed or preserved to eat as candy. This candy is also said to be a good remedy for indigestion. In large quantities, however, nutmeg can cause nausea, vomiting, and even stupor.

Oak || *Encino* || *Quercus sp.*

The leaves can be chewed, removed from the mouth, and applied to bites to stop itching. More often, however, the bark is dried, chopped and boiled for ten minutes, with the resulting liquid used as a gargle, douche, or enema for treating inflammation and skin problems, and as an astringent. It can also be brewed as a tea, and when taken this way, is said to cure diarrhea and also act as a diuretic. Oak leaves, when ground, are used as a snuff, and when boiled, as a blood tonic. In Mexico, two types of oak are referred to as *encino rojo*, while *encino blanco* and *robles* are larger trees.

Ocotillo, Candlewood || *Ocotillo* || *Fouqueria splendens*

Ocotillo treats bladder infections and stimulates tardy menstruation; not recommended for use during pregnancy. A tincture of the bark is used to treat varicose veins and hemorrhoids.

Olive || *Olivo* || *Olea europea*

The oil from crushed olives is used to treat cough. It is mixed with egg white to make a soothing ointment that is applied to the neck and chest, or is taken by itself, orally, a teaspoon at a time.

A spoonful of olive oil is also said to protect against intoxication. Modern studies have shown that this might indeed be so. The oil coats the stomach wall, inhibiting the penetration of the alcohol and at the same time, enabling enzymes to break the alcohol down before it can get into the bloodstream.

A spoonful of olive oil is also said to give high energy, much as a spoonful of honey does, by elevating the blood sugar. In addition, the leaves of the olive tree, and occasionally the bark, can be boiled to make a tea taken to rid the body of intestinal worms or to use as a wash for body sores and rashes.

Onion || *Cebolla* || *Allium cepa*

Raw onion is eaten to treat anemia, exhaustion, bronchial complaints, and gas. Onion that has been chopped and cooked in oil is fed to children to prevent scarlet fever and diphtheria. Crushed and decocted with honey, onion is taken as a tea for cough or sore throat.

Onion has a number of recorded external uses, too. It can be applied grated or in slices as a poultice over burns, bites, wounds, or even over joints which are troubled by rheumatic or arthritic pain. A roasted onion has great drawing power and is often applied, split and still hot, to boils. Mixed with hot vinegar, onion is used to make a chest compress to provide relief for those suffering from pneumonia.

Orange || *Naranja* || *Citrus aurantium*

A tea made from the leaves of the bitter orange (*naranja amarga*) is taken, variously, as a general tonic and calming agent, to aid digestion, to cure insomnia and even to alleviate heart palpitations. The fresh leaves, picked and boiled until the water is halved in volume, are also given to epileptics. Tea made from the peel and flowers is somewhat more potent and is taken to calm the nerves and, again, to combat sleeplessness. Too much, however, can have a toxic effect. Tea made from the bark of the bitter orange tree is taken several days in a row to stimulate the appetite. See Citron Flowers.

Oregano (Wild Marjoram) || *Orégano* || *Monarda sp.*

The leaves and heads of the flowers are dried and used to brew a tea taken to regulate menstruation, and relieve premenstrual tension and cramps. This tea induces perspiration and is said to loosen phlegm and soothe a sore throat and so is given to those with bronchitis. It is also used as a gargle. An even stronger oregano tea consumed before meals will supposedly expel intestinal worms. Mexican oregano, *Lippia sp.* is used as an antiseptic.

Oshá (Mountain Ginseng, Colorado Coughroot) || *Chuchapate* || *Ligusticum porteri*
The root of the oshá plant is used for a wide variety of ailments, including sore throats, gum irritations, flu and cold, coughs, and even the skin. On a more metaphysical level, oshá is believed to ward off evil spirits and curses.

Papaya || *Papaya* || *Carica papaya*
Papaya has been analyzed and is known to contain a soothing and healing enzyme, papain. The Indians of Mexico long ago discovered its properties and laid strips of the fruit upon infected wounds to cure them. Papaya is also applied in this way to jellyfish stings. In fact, a well-known meat tenderizer, which contains dried papaya, is often taken to the beach for this purpose. Papaya can be eaten, too, to cure indigestion. Its juice is soothing to those suffering from stomach ulcers.

Parsley || *Perejil* || *Petroselinum crispum*
This herb, too, has many and varied uses. Some herbalists, in fact, claim that regular consumption of a parsley tea will cure alcoholism. Still others say that it will dissolve gallstones when taken daily. More commonly, an infusion of fresh leaves makes a tea that is used to relieve indigestion or menstrual cramps. One less widely known use of parsley is to make a tea of crushed seeds to dry up a mother's milk after her baby is weaned. Externally, mashed parsley

leaves are applied to cuts, bleeding wounds, or insect stings. Similarly, the leaves can be packed in the nostril to stop nosebleed. The most controversial claim for parsley is that, eaten fresh each day, it will prevent cancer.

Passion Flower || *Passiflora, Passionaria* || *Passiflora sp.*
The stem and leaves are used as a sedative for insomnia and headaches.

Pecan || *Nuez, Pacanero* || *Carya illinoinensis*
The leaves are soaked in water overnight and the water is then strained and taken by people who are anemic. This is said to enrich their blood.

Pennyroyal || *Poleo de Casa, Poleo Chino* || *Hedeoma oblongifolium* (**commercial plant**: *H. pulegoides*)
A tea made of the dry leaves and flowering tips of the plant is reportedly a cold remedy, probably because it is diaphoretic. Externally, it is applied to insect bites to stop itching and promote healing. See Brook Mint.

Pepper Tree || *Pirul, Pirú* || *Schinus molle*
Boughs from this tree are said to have a magical effect. They are passed over the body of someone suffering from susto while the person performing the cure prays. But the effect of the pepper tree is also thought to be negative. It is said that those living in a house shaded by a pepper tree will be sterile, for instance. Of course, one of the most famous curanderos of all time, Niño Fidencio, sat under a pepper tree in the town of Espinazo to do much of his healing. As mentioned earlier in the text, the tree, El Pirulito, is much honored today and even has its own attendant. The leaves and fruit are used for wounds and toothaches.

Pine || *Pino* || *Pinus sp.*

Juice extracted from pine makes an excellent cough syrup as does pine sprig honey. These are also recommended treatments for bronchitis and chest infections. Externally, water in which pine needles have soaked overnight makes a bracing, and some say energy-restoring, bath water.

Piñon || *Trementina de Piñon* || *Pinus edulis*

A New Mexican remedy source specific to the state's native piñon pine (as opposed to the more generic listing immediately above), piñon pitch (*trementina*) is used to draw out slivers and splinters from the skin by placing it on the afflicted area while it is warm and thus liquid. When it dries, the pitch is pulled away from the skin and the splinter comes away with the pitch. It is also used to treat neuralgia, is sometimes rubbed on rheumatic joints, and is also used to draw pus from wounds.

Potato || *Papa* || *Solanum tuberosum*

The raw juice can be taken for relief from stomachache, diarrhea, and fluid retention. Slices of raw potato, too, can be placed on the temples to cure headache. Most often, however, grated potato is applied in poultice form to puffy eyelids, cracked skin, sunburn, or insect bites.

Prickly Pear Cactus || *Nopal* || *Opuntia sp.*

The Aztecs used the juice to treat burns, making it into a paste with egg yolks and honey. They also mixed it with maguey and drank it as a cure for hepatitis. The fruit of the prickly pear cactus, called the *tuna*, was also sliced in half and heated and placed on abscesses to draw out infection. Recently, the "*nopalitos*," or tender young plants, have been studied for their possible effect on reducing blood sugar or controlling diabetes.

Pumpkin || *Calabaza* || *Cucurbito pepo*

About a hundred pumpkin seeds (pepitas) are peeled and eaten raw to cure tapeworm. This should be done on an empty stomach. Extract can also be purchased for this purpose. Externally, pumpkin pulp can also be used as a cold poultice for headache and burns.

Red Dock || *Canaigre* || *Rumex hymenosepalus*

Canaigre is used as a mouthwash and to help stop bleeding in cuts and abrasions.

Red Pepper—see Cayenne Pepper.

Resurrection Plant || *Doradilla* || *Selaginella pilifera*

Five to six plants are boiled, strained, and sweetened for liver and kidney stones and irritations, intestinal parasites, and coughs. Some people place this plant in a glass of water and sprinkle the water at door entrances for good luck, health, and prosperity.

Rose of Castille || *Rosa de Castilla* || *Rosa sp., possibly R. centifolia*

A tea made from the flowers is given to children suffering from colic, diarrhea, and intestinal inflammation. It serves as a laxative. When cool it is also used as a wash for inflamed eyes. The powdered flowers are used for fever blisters (herpes).

Rosemary || *Romero* || *Rosmarinus officinalis*

This is another herb that is used as a cure for a wide variety of ills. The leaves are used often to make a tea to aid digestion and delayed menstruation, but it is also supposed to increase memory. The same tea, cooled, can be used as a skin wash to prevent wrinkles and blemishes and to erase freckles. Rosemary tea is also considered an excellent mouthwash and breath freshener. A very optimistic use is to rub a tincture of rosemary onto the head each day to prevent baldness. More reliably, the same tincture can be rubbed on painful joints and muscles.

Rue || *Ruda* || *Ruda sp.*

Rue tea, taken in small amounts, will stimulate menstruation. The same tea, again, in a small dose (one cup maximum) is recommended variously for relief from congestion, headache, nausea, fainting spells, difficult breathing, and stomach cramps. The tea, most herbals agree, should be taken without sugar.

Externally, rue tea can be used as a wash to kill body lice.

One book touts rue as a remedy for snakebite. It suggests that the plant be soaked in beer, then the beer applied directly to the bite. It further advises that the remainder be consumed.

For earache, a stem of rue wrapped in cotton and placed in the ear is said to erase the pain.

Sage || *Salvia* || *Salvia hispanica* or *tilliaefolia*, *Salvia sp.*

Sage is another of the wonder herbs, used for diverse ailments. It is best, most herbals advise, to use sage by itself, rather than in combination with other herbs.

Some of the medicinal uses include substitution of a sage tea for coffee to aid those with digestive problems. When added to a baby's formula, sage is said to fight diarrhea. It is also said to prevent tuberculosis, in children especially.

Sage, because it dries up all secretions, also provides a good tea for nursing women who wish to wean. In addition to depleting the milk supply, sage will slow the flow of mucous, perspiration, and saliva.

Sage tea is said to work against depression, too. When sage tea is cooled it makes an effective mouthwash, often used to cure gum disease. The same tea is antiseptic and destroys bacteria, thus providing a good soak for wounds.

Some lesser known uses are that sage can be smoked by asthmatics for relief, and that a sage leaf chewed before eating foods that tend "not to agree with" one will permit the user to eat the meal without ill effect.

Sagebrush (New Mexico), Taos Sage || *Chamiso Hediondo* || *Artemisia tridentata*

This New Mexico sage, as distinguished from the less clearly identified sages described above, is made into a cold tea for digestive problems. It is also used to alleviate colds and fevers, and for sweat baths to detoxify the body.

Sarsaparilla || *Raiz de Cocolmeca, Zarzaparilla* || *Smilax sp.*

The root is boiled in water and the resulting tea is then taken to purify the blood, thereby preventing or curing skin diseases and eruptions. The roots yield sarapogenin, which acts much like progesterone. The leaves and berries of the sarsaparilla plant are said to be a good antidote for poisons. Some herbals list this tea as a cure for syphilis as well as for hives, and claim that it can reduce heavy menstrual bleeding.

Scarlet Globemallow || *Yerba de la Negrita* || *Sphaeralcea coccinea*

The tea made from this prevalent New Mexico plant, famous for its distinctive orange-red blossoms, soothes sore throats; it is also used as a hair rinse to add body and for conditioning.

Sea Holly, Button Snakeroot || *Yerba del Sapo* || *Eryngium sp.*

The whole plant is brewed into a tea, preferably a decoction, which is taken to relieve water retention and kidney problems. The tea stimulates uterine contractions, too, and is often taken by women about to give birth, presumably to speed the delivery. Sea holly, because of its effect on the uterus, is also thought to be an aphrodisiac.

Seville Orange—see Orange.

Shaggy-Leafed Toadflax —see Toadflax.

Sorrell || *Acedera* || *Rumex acetosa*
Taken as a tea, Sorrell is a laxative. Cooked, it is used as a poultice, which will bring boils to a head.

Star Anise || *Anís Estrella* || *Illicum verum*
Taken as a tea it calm nerves; also aids sleep.

Stinging Nettle—see Nettle.

Stonecrop—see Houseleek.

Sunflower || *Girasol* || *Helianthus annuus*
A tincture is made to cure colds by mashing the stems and soaking them in alcohol for a month. The seeds, which are eaten, are said to have varied effects. Some eat them for potency. Another rumored use is to decrease fertility. Because they allegedly contract the uterus, sunflower seeds are also said to cause abortion.

Sweet Basil—see Basil.

**Tapacola || *Salvia de Monte, Hierba del Soldado* ||
*Waltheria americana***
This plant, as one of its common names (tapacola) indicates, is used for diarrhea and to clean wounds.

Tepezcohuite || *Tepezcohuite || Mimosa tenuiflora*

Tepezcohuite is thought to promote healing for skin conditions such as burns. It has no known English name that I have discovered, although it is known as the "skin tree" in Mexico. It apparently has rather potent skin regenerative properties and promotes cellular regeneration, which would account for its reputation for combating aging and helping to heal burns. The name seems to refer to both the tree and to the bark, which is the part used for treatment of skin conditions.

Thyme || *Tomillo || Thymus vulgaris*

Thyme is thought to induce abortion. Less dramatically, a tea made of thyme is said to eliminate phlegm and postnasal drip. Thyme tea is thought to have a different effect depending upon its temperature, and thus a cold thyme tea is taken for headache relief, while a hot brew is consumed to induce sleep and to ward off nightmares. Hot thyme tea is reportedly good to use as a remedy for stomach cramps and diarrhea.

But thyme can be used externally, too, and in fact, has been found to contain an antibacterial substance. One can use it on sores and insect bites, or brew a very strong solution to fumigate and repel insects. Oil of thyme has strong germicidal qualities.

Toadflax || *Hojas de Callito, Linaria || Linaria vulgaris*

Press the flowering stems until liquid is extracted and use as a mouthwash, one herbal advises. Another suggests that you brew a tea from the stems when the plant is in flower and use it as a liver stimulant and hepatic remedy.

Toronjil—see Lemon Balm.

Tree Gloxina || *Tlanchichinole* || *Kohleria deppeana*
This plant is used for kidney problems, digestive disorders, and diarrhea. Externally it is used to clean wounds, vaginal infections, and hemorrhoids.

Tree Spinach || *La Chaya* || *Cnidoscolus chayamansa*
La chaya is currently being used as a food supplement because of its high iron, calcium, vitamin A, and vitamin C content. It is also used as a laxative and a diuretic. In the Southwest, people have cooked it and boiled the leaves in order to treat diabetes. Tree spinach has been used as food for thousands of years by aboriginal Americans. La chaya must be cooked to be taken safely. Fresh leaves contain toxic hydrocyanic glycosides, which are rendered inactive by cooking.

Trumpet Flower, Yellowbells || *Tronadora* || *Tecoma stans*
Dried *tronadora* is used to control diabetes, to prevent kidney problems, and to treat fevers. It is also used for hangovers.

Uva Ursi—see Bearberry.

Valerian, Garden Heliotrope || *Raíz de Valeriana* || *Valeriana sp.*
Only the root of this potent plant is used. Its results are rumored to be varied and include inducing abortion, serving as an anaphrodisiac, and curing alcoholism. One proven effect is that it is a powerful sedative and antispasmodic. It is also used for insomnia and nervousness.

The root is ground into a powder and mixed with water—never boiled—and taken for nervousness, cramps, or insomnia. Valerian should not be used regularly because it can cause depression. Cats love valerian powder and will react to it much as they do to catnip.

The fresh root is less odorific than the dried, though the latter is more frequently available. Valerian powder can also be applied dry to sores and abscesses.

Vanilla || *Vainilla* || *Vanilla planifolia* or *Vanilla fragrans*
Sweetened and mixed with water or milk, vanilla is variously listed as an aid to digestion, a stimulant, an antispasmodic, and an emmenagogue, e.g., a substance that stimulates menstrual flow.

Vervain || *Verbena* || *Verbena sp.*
Tea made from the leaves of vervain reduces fever and induces perspiration. It is taken for colds and the flu. The same tea rubbed on the scalp is said to promote hair growth.

Violet || *Violeta* || *Viola sp.*
A mild decoction is taken for headache, as a sedative, or even a remedy for cough or cold. The fresh leaves, when crushed, are also applied to cracked nipples or gouty limbs. A decoction made of violet root is emetic, meaning that it can be used to induce vomiting when that is desired—when a poison has been ingested, for instance. Sometimes a candy is made from violets.

Walnut || *Nogal* || *Juglans regia, J. major*
A decoction made of the leaves of this tree is a disinfectant and can be applied to wounds and sores. The bark is a laxative and the leaves are used for diarrhea. Both the leaves and roots are taken for arthritis. It is also said to have insect repelling capabilities and is used to bathe humans and pets.

Watercress || *Berro* || *Nasturtium officinale*
This herb is always used fresh and uncooked, though it should be washed well since it tends to attract dogs that use it to mark their

territories. Chewed, watercress is anti-inflammatory and will stop gums from bleeding. Crushed, the extract thus produced is consumed for ailments as diverse as diabetes, anemia, and bronchitis. Watercress, which contains manganese, is said to lower blood sugar.

Wild Marjoram—see Oregano.

Willow, especially White Willow || *Sáuce, Sáuz, Jara, Jarita* || *Salix sp.*
The bark contains salycin, which is like aspirin. The powder from ground willow bark is anti-inflammatory and analgesic and is taken in capsules or mixed with wine to reduce fever or to relieve the pain of headaches, rheumatism, or arthritis. Tea made from willow bark is also used to combat bladder infections. Boiled with borax or boric acid, willow is a good antiseptic wash.

Wormwood || *Agenjo, Ajenjo* || *Artemisia mexicana*
As a bitter tea, *agenjo* stimulates the digestive system and improves appetite. Also used for liver disorders. Combined with other bitter herbs, it can be used in baths to relieve arthritis and skin rashes, or for gall bladder illness. In some regions, wormwood is also referred to as *estafiate*. See Mugwort (Western).

Yam Bean || *Jicama, Xiquima* || *Pachyrhizus erosus*
The seeds in tincture are applied to the head to cure dandruff.

Yarrow || *Milenrama, Plumajillo* || *Achillea lanulosa*
Yarrow is another plant supposedly used to induce abortion. In fact, it has a multiplicity of reported uses.

Externally, a tea brewed from yarrow is said to be an insect repellent which can be splashed over the body. The same tea is also used as a skin lotion. Fresh yarrow leaves, applied to a wound, will allegedly stop even a profuse flow of blood and will also stimulate clotting. A poultice of dried leaves will, it is said, disinfect and promote healing.

Taken internally, yarrow is thought to have the same effect, supposedly decreasing the menstrual flow and stopping internal hemorrhage. It is also taken to decrease the likelihood of varicose veins and to banish leg cramps. The same tea is a mild laxative and, some say, stomach tonic.

Yerba Anís—see Marigold (Sweet).

Yerba Buena (Hierba Buena)—see Mint.

Yerba de la Negrita—see Scarlet Globemallow.

**Yerba Mansa (Swamp Root) || *Yerba Mansa* ||
*Anemopsis californica***
As a tea, this New Mexican herbal remedy is used for stomach disorders and as a gargle. It is also used in liniments for arthritis and rheumatism since it is anti-inflammatory, and in powdered form for hemorrhoids and abrasions. The root and leaves can also be taken as a tea for rheumatoid arthritis.

**Yerba Santa (Mountain Balm, Holly Herb) || *Yerba Santa* ||
*Eriodictyon angustifolia, E. californicum***
This herbal remedy of New Mexico is used for various respiratory problems, to clear various passages (sinuses, bronchial paths, lungs) of phlegm. Prepared as a tea, it apparently is also used as a diuretic and for pain affecting the urethra. Another plant, *hoja santa* (*Piper auritum*) is also used for various respiratory problems.

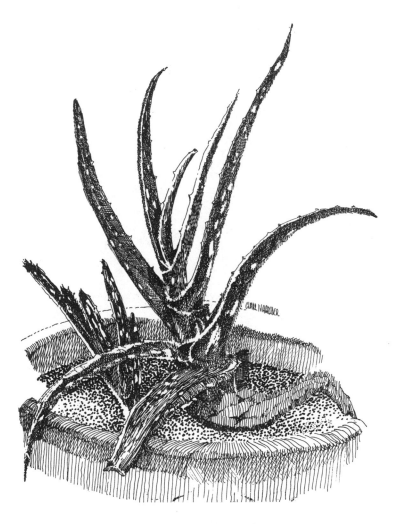

Figure 20: Aloe vera (zabila) is known to
alleviate burns and skin irritations.

Index

ritual sacrifice and, 8; rituals of, 6, 8, 21–22, 125; roots of, 5, 66, 85–88; spells and hexes and, 18, 20; spiritual aspects of, 6, 21, 23–25, 30, 32–33; supernatural and, 10–11; symbolic colors and, 31; symbolic objects and, 21; theory of the humors and, 5, 88; three levels of, 5–6. *See also* green medicine; herbal medicine

Curanderismo (the book), 6, 70

Curanderismo: Mexican-American Folk Psychiatry, 70

Curanderos/as, 4, 5; Anglo, 62; apprenticeship and, 10; black, 18; Catholic Church and, 61; formal medicine and, 60; God and, 10, 21; healthcare and, 66; modern, 11–12, 59–64; patient and, 30; payment for, 10–11, 41, 61; power of, 58–59; *recetas* of, 60; state of consciousness of, 9; status of, 30; the supernatural and, 11; white, 18

Cures: Apostles' Creed and, 27; brooms and, 24–25, 27, 32; eggs and (*see* eggs); expectation of, 84; holy water and, 25; rituals and, 21–25; symbolic objects and, 21–25

Cuts. *See* abrasions; wounds

Cystitis, 136, 141–42, 145

Damian. See *Damiana de California*

Damiana de California (Damian), 98, 101, 128

Dandelion. See *Diente de León*

Dandruff, 132, 157. *See also* ·hair

Dare, Helen, 60

Davidow, Jolie, 105

De la Cruz-Badiano Aztec

herbal of 1552, 106–7

Delphinium (Larkspur). See *Espuela de Caballero*

Demulcents, 99

Depression, 136, 141, 152, 155

Desasombro (high level of *susto*), 13, 16; treatment for, 27

Diabetes, 133, 155, 157; controlling, 140, 150, 155; Type II, 123

Diaphoretics, 99

Diarrhea: treatment for, 122, 127, 137, 142, 145, 149, 150, 151, 153, 154, 155, 156

Diente de León (Dandelion), 128–29

Digestion: aids for, 125, 126, 130, 133, 141, 146, 150, 156; problems, 151, 152, 155; stimulation for, 157. *See also* indigestion; stomach

Diphtheria, 146

Discovering Folklore Through Community Resources, 24–25, 71; treatments in, 27

Disinfectants, 127; for wounds, 128, 156

Diuretics: herbs that are, 99, 128, 129, 130, 133, 134, 135, 136, 145, 155, 158. *See also* water retention

Dodson, Ruth, 18, 26, 38, 39, 71

Don Pedrito Jaramillo, 18, 22, 37, 61, 71; as folk saint, 36, 46; cures of, 25–26, 39–40, 60; life and miracles of, 38–41; *Los Olmos* and, 38; psychic powers of, 39; *recetas* of, 60–61; Severiano Barrera and, 41; shrine of, 38

Don Pedrito Jaramillo: Curandero, 71

Don, the, 10

Doradilla (Resurrection Plant), 150

Dysentery, 121, 140, 142

Dysmenorrhea (*see also* menstruation), 127, 130, 147

Earaches, 123, 126, 143

Edema, 129. *See also* water retention

Eggs: *empacho* and, 26; use of, 6, 8, 21–23, 24, 64. See also *curanderismo*

El Niño. *See* Niño Fidencio

El Proyecto Comprender script, 58–59

Elder Flower. *See* Saúco

Elm. See *Olmo*

Embrujada (bewitched), 18

Emetics, 99, 156

Emmenagogues, 99, 156

Emollients, 99

Emotions: anger. *See muína*; depression, 136, 141, 152, 155; fright. *See susto*; health and, 12; nerves. *See nerves*

Empacho (stomach blockage), 13; herbs for, 135; prepackaged remedies for, 95–96; symptoms of, 15; theory of humors and, 15; treatment for, 26. *See also* stomach

Encino (Oak), 98, 145; *blanco*, 145; *robles*, 145; *rojo*, 145

Enebro (*Tascate*) (Juniper), 135–36

Envidia (envy), 13, 17

Envy. See *envidia*

Epazote (Mexican Tea, Wormseed), 99, 141

Epazote de Zorillo, 141

Epilepsy, 135, 142, 146

Espanto (serious loss of spirit), 13, 16; causes of, 16

Espiritistas (mediums), 10, 81

Espliego (*Alhucema, Lavanda*) (Lavender), 136–37

Espuela de Caballero (*Delfinio*), 129

Estafiate (Western Mugwort), 142. See also *Agenjo*

Estramonio (*Tolache, Floripondio*) (Jimson Weed), 92

Eucalipto (Eucalyptus), 92, 123, 130

Lettuce. See *Lechuga*
Lice: body, 129, 135, 151
Lily of the Valley. See *Lirio de Los Valles*
Limón, 101, 137. *See also* Lemons
Linden Flower. See *Flor de Tila*
Liniments: herbal, 99, 128
Lirio de Los Valles (Lilly of the Valley), 138
Liver, 128–29; disorders, 140, 150, 157; stimulants, 154
Longevity, 120
Los Remedios, 105
Luck: belief in, 33; incense and, 33; questions about, 35

Magic: black, 10; white, 10
Magnolia. See *Flor de Corazón*
Maguey (Agave) (Century Plant, Mescal), 89, 125, 149
Mal aire (respiratory infection) (*see also* coughs; flu), 13, 16; teas for, 148, 156; treatment for, 27, 130, 137, 141, 144, 146, 147, 152, 158
Mal de ojo (evil eye), 3, 13–14; Apostles' Creed and, 23; preventatives for, 31, 132; treatment for, 29
Mal puesto, 13, 17
Malaria: herbs for, 124–25; quinine and, 80
Maleficio, 13, 17
Mallow. See *Malva*
Malva (Mallow; Musk Mallow), 138–39, 143
Manzanilla (Chamomile), 3–4, 87, 88, 99; introduction from Spain of, 88; *te de*, 60; uses for, 125
Manzanitas, 121
María, 61–62
Marigold (Sweet). See *Pericón*
Marigold. See *Caléndula*
Marijuana, 92, 139–40
Mariquilla (Goldenrod), 133

Marjoram. See *Mejorana*
Marrubio Concha (Horehound), 133
Materia Medica, 81
Measles, 122
Medicinal Plants of the Mountain West, 104–105
Medicine: Arabic, 85. *See also curanderismo*; formal medicine; green medicine; herbal medicine
Mejorana (Marjoram), 140
Memory, 151
Menopause: difficulty with, 142
Menstruation, 127, 130, 134; excessive bleeding and, 144, 152, 158; inducing, 130, 133, 141, 145, 151, 156; painful, 136, 137, 142, 147; PMS and, 130, 147; regulating, 147
Mercados, 91
Mesquite, 140
Mexican Day Flower. See *Yerba del Pollo*
Mexican Quinine. See *Palo Amargo*
Mexican Tarragon, 119
Mexican Tea (Wormseed). See *Epazote*
Mexican yam, 105
Mexico: Indians of, 85–86; traditional medicine in, 88, 102–3. *See also* Aztecs
Mexico's Ancient and Native Remedies, 6, 105
Meyer, G, Kenneth Blum, and John G. Cull, 105–6
Michener, James, 36
Migraines, 130. *See also* headaches
Milenrama (*Plumajillo*) (Yarrow), 157–58
Mint (*Yerba Buena*), 4, 90, 98, 99
Modern medicine: *curanderismo* and, 12, 65–68, 82, 85. *See also* healthcare
Moja de Guaco, 122
Monkshood (Wolfsbane). See *Acónito*

Moon: beliefs about, 31–32; bewitchment by, 32
Moore, Michael, 104–5
Mormon Tea. See *Cañutillo*
Morning Glory. See *Tumbavaquero*
Mostaza (Mustard), 144
Mountain Balm. See *Yerba Santa*
Mouthwashes, 150, 151, 152, 154. *See also* gargles
Mucous membranes, 139
Mugwort (Mountain). See *Altamisa*
Mugwort (Western). See *Estafiate*
Muína (rage), 13, 17; treatment for, 28 *See also* emotions
Mulberry. See *Corteza de Mora*
Mullein. See *Gordolobo*
Mumps, 139
Musk Mallow. See *Malva*
Mustard. See *Mostaza*

Naranja (Orange), 146; bitter, 146
Native American: herbal lore, 85
Nausea: treatment for, 127, 132–33, 141, 145, 151
Nerves: calming the, 125, 137, 138, 141, 146, 153, 155; disorders of the, 142
Nettle (Stinging Nettle). See *Ortiga Mayor*
Neuralgia, 149
Newbury, Henrietta, 71
Nightmares, 154 *See also* insomnia
Niño Fidencio, 10, 18, 43; as folk saint, 46; burial site of, 45; cures of, 44; death of, 46; *El Camino de Penitencia* and, 45; *El Charquito* and, 45; *El Pirulito* and, 45; Pepper Tree and, 148–49; pilgrimages to burial site of, 46, 82; shrines to, 45. See also *Fidencistas*